THE
COMPLETE GUIDE TO
DIGESTIVE
HEALTH

By the same author:
THE SALT-WATCHER'S GUIDE
BRITTLE BONES AND THE CALCIUM CRISIS

THE
COMPLETE GUIDE TO
DIGESTIVE HEALTH

END POOR DIGESTION
WITH THIS SELF-HELP PLAN

Kathleen Mayes

THORSONS PUBLISHING GROUP

First published 1990

British Library Cataloguing in Publication Data

Mayes, Kathleen
  The complete guide to digestive health.
  1. Man. Stomach. Diseases
  I. Title
  616.3'3

ISBN 0-7225-2175-8

Published by Thorsons Publishers Limited, Wellingborough, Northamptonshire NN8 2RQ, England

Typeset by Harper Phototypesetters Limited, Northampton, England
Printed in Great Britain by Mackays, Chatham, Kent

10 9 8 7 6 5 4 3 2 1

Contents

Note to the reader

This information is presented not with the intention of diagnosing or prescribing, but to help the reader cooperate with his or her doctor in a mutual desire to improve and maintain health.

No responsibility is assumed on the part of the author, the publisher, or the distributors of this work. It is not the purpose of this publication to replace the services of a doctor, nor is it the purpose to guarantee any medicinal or nutritional preparation or the effectiveness thereof.

Before beginning any changes in your diet, it is recommended that you should consult your doctor.

Any use of brand names in this guide is for identification only, and does not imply endorsement or otherwise by the author.

PART ONE

An overview

Introduction

Humans can now walk on the moon, dive the ocean depths and travel at supersonic speed, but are still only equipped with basically the same system of body nourishment and waste excretion that our prehistoric ancestors had 100,000 years ago.

Human culture and behaviour has evolved significantly: communication has gone from primitive sounds to a profusion of languages to high-tech computers and instant telecommunications. Society has changed from small family groups in caves to sprawling mega-cities around the globe. Only a tiny minority continue the hunter-gatherer lifestyle of early peoples; most of us depend on food supplies in supermarkets, and our only exercise is walking from dining table to TV set. But what of our bodies? The physical evolution of human anatomy has been less significant, yet we are threatened by an abundance of food, the wrong type of food, and decreasing physical activity, combining to break down our digestive system.

Ancient hunting-gathering societies were no healthier than our own. Undoubtedly, many of our primitive ancestors were victims of famine, seasonal malnutrition, poisonous plants, contaminated food and water, and severe vitamin deficiencies, but in later times, agriculture provided a food supply that was more dependable. Then dairying and cattle-herding increased the sources of fats in the diet, and reduced the quantity of non-nutritive fibre. Tobacco was nonexistent in most of the Old World, although some pre-agricultural people probably chewed tobacco. Alcohol was probably only available seasonally: natural fermentation produced drinks such as beer of relatively low potency, but there was no distillation of spirits.

Today, the digestive system faces many challenges. We have an overabundance of food and the ability to afford it. Much of it is processed and highly-refined – loaded with fats, sweeteners and refined flours – and lacking in bulk. Advertising encourages overeating, and promotes smoking and drinking as glamorous. Exercise is minimized: manual labour is decreasing; 'labour saving' reduces the need to move your body; driving replaces walking, even for short distances; sports are enjoyed more from the stands than on the playing fields; homes are heated with the flick of a switch or thermostat instead of the swing of an axe. Stress today is increased by overcrowded cities, overwork, international tensions, or problems closer to home, yet many gastrointestinal reflexes were designed for readiness to fight or flee predators. No wonder the digestive tract rebels.

Except for chewing and swallowing, you probably don't give much thought to your digestive system. It is completely automatic. Hastily stuffing down food, you eat on the run, washing down each mouthful with hot drinks, fizzy drinks or alcohol. You have a hectic pace at work, a quick cigarette, a rushed lunch, then cope with problems around the house after work. And if your system kicks back at the onslaught, you get surprised, annoyed or impatient. But it has been affronted by what you have made it go through. This complex collection of organs and chemicals gives pleasure when it works properly, and misery when it goes wrong. Now and then you are acutely aware of its existence.

So what *is* good digestion? It is taking in the right type of food, the right amount of food suitable for your age, the breaking down of the food, both physically and chemically, into separate nutrient components that the body can use. It is the absorption of that food to provide new cells, maintain tissue, provide energy calories for keeping warm, calories for activities, and the storage of moderate fat reserves for future bodily needs. And it is the gentle regular elimination of waste products – indigestible fibres from foods, discarded cells, and gases produced by the chemical action of some foods.

Your digestive tract is constantly undergoing change, gradually evolving as you age and with the foods that challenge it. From the first time that a baby's lips seek nourishment from breast or bottle to the last spoonfuls of food taken by an elderly person, the gastrointestinal tract changes physically and chemically, with the foods it can accept and properly assimilate. And if you don't recognize that a change has occurred, instead of digestion you have indigestion.

Patients fill doctors' surgeries seeking relief from stomach pain, chemists and drug stores do a brisk business in prescription drugs, non-prescription medicines and remedies for heartburn, cramps, constipation and haemorrhoids. It's a multi-million pound industry. But before rushing to the medicine cabinet or to the doctor for a pill, you can often find solutions in other ways. In some cases, a simple change of diet or lifestyle is all you need to put things right.

The next chapter gives a simplified explanation of the complex mechanisms that make up normal digestion. Part Two shows some of the habits of eating or lifestyle that frequently cause trouble to the digestive tract, and how they may be minimized or avoided. Part Three describes the most common problems: preventive action to avoid the problems in the first place, prescriptions, alternative solutions, when to recognize the need for a physician, and what the doctor can do for you.

A good working system is up to you. Read on and find out how to keep your system healthy!

CHAPTER 1

How should the system work?

The warm fragrance of freshly-baked bread wafts down the street from the baker's – a golden-brown apple pie scents the kitchen – a savoury aroma and sizzle comes from bacon under the grill. Is your mouth already watering in anticipation? Your digestion is working even *before* you put any food into your mouth!

Appetite is regulated by a delicate mechanism in the *hypothalamus*, a small cluster of specialized cells at the base of the brain. When you sniff aromas through your nostrils, or receive them between nasal passages and mouth when eating or drinking, olfactory receptors convey messages to the *limbic* region of the brain, which tells you whether or not food is pleasurable. The limbic system activates the hypothalamus (the master switchboard for the pituitary gland) to stimulate the production of hormones controlling appetite, body temperature, metabolism, caloric levels, and more. The *appestat*, or appetite regulator, monitors levels of fat, protein, sugar and oxygen in the blood, and reacts to chemical signals from the digestive system.

Food and drink travels through about 9 metres (30 feet) of internal channels, along the route known as the alimentary canal, or the gastrointestinal (GI) tract, where food substances are churned and mixed with saliva, powerful acid secretions and enzymes. (See Figure 1.)

The GI tract is a continuous tube going from the mouth to the oesophagus (gullet), the stomach, small intestine, colon, rectum and anus. It has four basic functions: to break foods down physically into small pieces, to reduce them chemically to simple components (sugars, fatty acids and amino acids), to absorb these particles into the bloodstream, and to release and get rid of any residue that is unusable by the body.

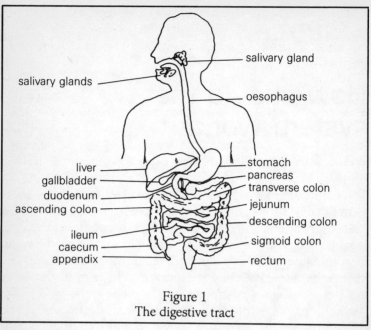

Figure 1
The digestive tract

The teeth

Digestion begins in the mouth where food is broken up by chewing. Teeth are set in both upper and lower jaws, held in place by the gums which are dense fibrous tissues technically called *gingivae*. The teeth are equipment for cutting, tearing and grinding food that is not already liquid, with the food being moved about by the muscular movements of the tongue.

The tongue

The tongue is a muscular organ that moves portions of food around the mouth and towards the throat, it provides a sense of taste and helps us to speak. The sense of taste is fully developed at birth.

Sensations of taste arise from the activity of groups of specialized cells on the tongue's upper surface. These epithelial cells are commonly called taste-buds, of which the average adult has a few thousand. Babies and children have greater numbers of taste-buds than adults, at the back of the throat, the underside of the tongue and the inner surface of the cheeks. The number of taste-buds diminishes gradually with age, especially after the age of 45 years. The cells that compose a taste-bud have a life of about ten days and are continuously being regrown – which is fortunate when you burn your tongue!

There are four basic taste sensations: sweet, bitter, sour and salty. There may be two more: the metallic, when for instance the mouth bleeds or when it is in contact with iron or copper; and the alkaline or soapy taste. The four principal tastes can be sensed all over the tongue, but the taste-buds most sensitive to sweetness are along the front tip, sourness along the sides, saltiness along the front edge and bitterness across the back of the tongue. (See Figure 2.)

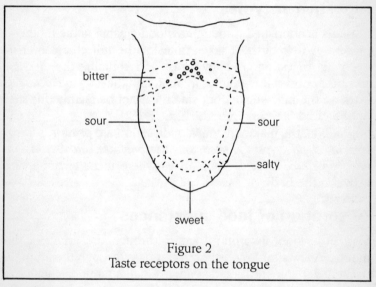

Figure 2
Taste receptors on the tongue

Tasting food is a joint effort of taste and smell, with smell the dominant partner. The tongue gives us the ability to determine a few different chemicals, but the nose with its olfactory cells can detect the presence of and differentiate between hundreds of different substances – a relic of the importance of smell among mammals.

Saliva

A healthy mouth always has *saliva*, a colourless liquid secretion from salivary glands in various positions around the mouth.

Saliva (or spittle or spit) has many components, among the most important of which is *mucin* that lubricates the inside of the mouth, and moistens and softens food going to the stomach. A human produces about half a litre to a litre (1 to 2 pints) of saliva each day, even when not actually chewing. Salivary glands are supplied with nerve endings that are so sensitive that even the thought or smell of a pleasing food morsel can trigger them into action and send forth increased amounts of saliva – hence the phenomenon we call 'mouth watering'. Another component of saliva is *ptyalin*, an enzyme that converts dietary starches into the sugars *maltose* and *dextrose*.

Digestive enzymes

A foetus is nourished through its bloodstream via the mother's placenta. After birth, it takes time for the full changeover to intestinal digestion. A baby's stomach contains the enzyme *rennin* to convert the proteins in milk, and the enzyme *lactase* to work on the milk sugars; but starch cannot be readily digested until a child is several months old.

In adults, the major enzymes of digestion are *ptyalin, pepsin, trypsin, chymotrypsin, lipase, amylase, maltase, sucrase, lactase and peptidase.* Table 1 summarizes where these enzymes are active in the body.

Absorption of food substances

Very little food absorption occurs through the lining of the mouth. A few simple substances can pass through the lining of the stomach into the bloodstream in small quantities, including water, alcohol, sugars, water-soluble minerals, water-soluble vitamins (for instance, vitamin C and the B vitamins, except B_{12}).

Most nutrient absorption occurs through the walls of the small intestine, including water, alcohol, starches and sugars (in the form of galactose, glucose and fructose), minerals, water-soluble vitamins, fat-soluble vitamins, proteins (in the form of peptides and amino acids), and fats in the form of glycerol and fatty acids.

But if foods pass through the GI tract too quickly, absorption can be considerably reduced, resulting in mineral and vitamin deficiencies. This occurs, for example, with overuse of laxatives and too much fibre in the diet.

TABLE 1
MAJOR DIGESTIVE ENZYMES AND
WHERE THEY ARE ACTIVE

Food Component	Mouth	Stomach	Intestine
Milk protein		RENNIN (in infants only) to produce peptides	PEPTIDASES to produce amino acids
Lactose (sugar found in milk)			LACTASE splits it to galactose and glucose
Starch	PTYALIN (from saliva) converts some to maltose and dextrose. AMYLASE converts to maltose	AMYLASE (from pancreas) converts to maltose	MALTASE converts maltose to glucose
Sucrose			SUCRASE converts it to glucose and fructose
Fats			LIPASE (from pancreas and intestine) converts to fatty acids
Proteins		PEPSIN to peptides. TRYPSIN and CHYMO-TRYPSIN (from pancreas) to peptides and amino acids	PEPTIDASES to amino acids

Along the GI tract

Once food is moistened, chewed and reduced to a semi-liquid, the tongue rolls it into a ball and coaxes it to the back of the mouth in the act of swallowing. At this point the voluntary portion of digestion stops, and everything afterwards should proceed automatically.

When swallowing, the *uvula*, hanging from the soft palate, moves up to close off the nasal passages. From the *pharynx*, two tubes lead from the throat into the lower part of the body: the *oesophagus* (gullet) carries food to the stomach, and the *trachea* carries air to the lungs. A flap of tissue, the *epiglottis*, moves into position, according to whatever enters the pharynx, allowing air to the trachea, or food and drink into the oesophagus.

The oesophagus

This section is about 24cm (9½ inches) long, and food takes just a few seconds to go down, depending on whether you have swallowed a liquid or a solid. Muscles of the oesophagus that encircle the tube perform *peristalsis*, which is a squeezing action to propel food and drink down to the stomach. At the end of the oesophagus is the circular sphincter muscle called the *lower oesophageal sphincter*. When food approaches, this muscle relaxes to allow food into the stomach, and then constricts quickly to prevent material in the stomach from backing up. This sphincter is important because pressure in the stomach is normally higher than in the oesophagus.

The stomach

It is essentially a bag of muscle and other tissue that serves as a holding tank where food is further churned and mashed by its rhythmic contractions. The stomach size and shape varies in each person and is capable of containing approximately a litre (quart) of food or liquid, although the wall of the stomach is very elastic, and it can expand tremendously to hold a much larger volume or contract according to the amount it contains. The wall has four layers consisting of muscles, nerve fibres, blood vessels, and glands: *parietal cells* manufacturing hydrochloric acid, *chief cells* providing *pepsin*, and *endocrine glands*. Parietal cells in gastric mucosa number about one thousand million in men and 800 million in women. The *vagus* nerve and its branches run from the base of the brain to the oesophagus, stomach, and liver; in the stomach, it controls parietal cells and stomach movements (*motility*). The presence of food stimulates a hormone, *gastrin*, secreted from the stomach's *antrum* section, that signals the release of pepsin enzyme and hydrochloric acid, in the digestive factory. The inner surface of the stomach wall, the *gastric mucosa*, completely replaces itself about once every three days, with millions of cells continuously being sloughed off and replaced. Glands secrete chemicals used during digestion, and a *mucous barrier* that protects the stomach wall from its own chemicals.

Gastric juice is like a recipe with a number of ingredients that should be present in the right amounts for the formula to work. The two main constituents of gastric juice, hydrochloric acid and pepsin, work on food material as it enters the stomach, and literally cause it to disintegrate.

Depending on which type it is, food usually remains in the stomach for three to four hours before passing on; fats can remain for up to six hours. While food is stored in the stomach, the peristaltic contractions of the stomach walls mix the food thoroughly with the digestive juices. Although television advertisers often give the impression that stomach contents should not be acid at all, the acidity of stomach juice is entirely natural and beneficial.

After it is thoroughly mashed and mixed, the food material – now called *chyme*, moves to the lower section of the stomach referred to as the *antrum* and then through the *pylorus*, a muscular valve at the lower end of the stomach, into the small intestine. The pylorus allows only a small amount of chyme through at a time because the small intestine can handle only so much. Carbohydrates, which require less work from the digestive system, move through the pylorus faster than proteins and fats.

The small intestine

The small intestine is named for its small diameter rather than for its length of 6 to 6.5 metres (20 to 22 feet). At the point where it leaves the stomach, the small intestine is only about 4 to 5cm (1½ to 2 inches) in diameter. There are three sections: the *duodenum*, the *jejenum* and the *ileum*. The duodenum is about 25 to 28cm (10 to 11 inches) long. In the duodenum, the acidity of the chyme is subjected to juices from the pancreas and bile from the liver. These juices neutralize the hydrochloric acid and cause a further breakdown of carbohydrates, proteins and fats. The final digestion of chyme and the absorption of nutrients takes place in the jejenum and ileum.

The *pancreas* is the second largest gland in the body and weighs about 85 grams (3 ounces). Pancreatic juice contains the enzyme amylase for starch-splitting, and lipase for fat-splitting, plus trypsin and chymotrypsin.

The *liver* is the body's largest gland, weighing up to 2kg (3 to 4 pounds). It is the chief chemical factory or junction box of the body, capable of many different chemical reactions. The liver secretes a yellowish juice called *gall* or *bile*, and the bile is conducted towards the duodenum by means of the *hepatic duct*. Bile is continuously being secreted by the liver, but between meals it is stored in a special pear-shaped sac called the *gallbladder*. When food arrives in the duodenum, the muscular wall of the gallbladder contracts and bile is forced through a passage called the *cystic duct*, into the *common bile duct*. Bile contains no enzymes, but has compounds called *bile salts*, important for breaking up fat into small globules that mix with water for more efficient fat digestion. Bile contains a number of waste products that are excreted via the liver and the gastrointestinal (GI) tract, for instance bile pigments that remain after natural processing of red blood cells, and it is these bile pigments that give the reddish-brown colour to stools when they are finally eliminated from the body.

Absorption in the small intestine takes place through the actions of tiny hair-like projections called *villi* that line the intestines to give the inner lining a velvety appearance. After the chyme has completed its passage through the small intestine, 95 per cent of the nutrients have been absorbed. Enzymes in the villi go to work breaking down protein, fats and carbohydrates. The absorptive surface of your small intestine is as large as a singles tennis court. This large surface area is created by folds of villi and microvilli lining the intestinal wall, and serves to extend the surface of the intestine and increase absorption. At the base of each villus is a group of cells that secrete still another fluid, the intestinal juice to break down food fragments: peptidases to break down proteins to the ultimate building blocks, the amino acids.

The remainder is sent on to the large intestine, or colon, which takes care of the absorption of water and such substances as sodium, potassium, chloride and bicarbonate.

The colon

Food now enters the last major portion of the alimentary canal, the large intestine (often called the *colon*). At the beginning of the large intestine is a blind alley called the *caecum*, and attached to the caecum is a worm-shaped appendage about 5 to 10cm (2 to 4 inches) long, the *appendix* which has no known function.

The colon is about 1.5m (5 feet) long, 6.3cm (2½ inches) wide, and divided into four regions: first the *ascending* colon, which lies on the right side of your abdomen; then making an abrupt turn at the liver, the tube becomes the *transverse* colon. A downward turn at the spleen is the beginning of the *descending* colon, which passes into the pelvic area and forms an S-shaped curve called the *sigmoid* colon.

By now, digestion is finished, as there is no digestion to speak of in the large intestine. But the absorption of water continues to form a semi-solid waste for excretion. The body has used water lavishly in its maintenance of mucosa and various digestive secretions along the way, but as water is subtracted, the contents of the large intestine become increasingly solid, although of course still soft.

The rectum

This is a vertical column of about 10 or 12cm (4 or 5 inches) from the sigmoid colon to the *anus* where body wastes leave through two *anal sphincter muscles*. The natural wave-like muscular action of the rectum eliminates the faeces. Defecation is usually accompanied or preceded by the escape of gases formed by bacterial action in the large intestine: carbon dioxide from fermented carbohydrates and nitrogen- and sulphur-containing residues from animal proteins and fats.

Faeces' solids consist of indigestible food residues, cellulose and discarded cell tissue. At least half of the stool is composed of bacteria.

Microflora and bacteria

The lower reaches of the intestine and colon normally harbour a resident population of healthy bacteria numbering in the millions – apart from the occasional temporary trouble-makers. Resident microorganisms originate from food, water, air, dust and saliva, and enter the digestive tract via the mouth at some time or another. There is little colonization of microorganisms in the stomach because of the strong germicidal action of gastric juices, and many bacteria are killed as they enter the stomach. The further away from the stomach, the greater the chance of the growth of bacteria, so the colon supports teeming populations of microorganisms.

The food we eat fosters colonies of a wide range of flora, including *Lactobacilli*, *Streptococci*, *Staphylococci*, coliform bacteria, and yeasts. The mixture of flora varies with each person, depending on the composition of digestive juices, food, and the kinds of antibodies that have developed. Some of these organisms are not mere parasites, because they pay a kind of 'rent' by synthesizing vitamins such as K, B_2, thiamine, riboflavin, folic acid and biotin. The population of normal intestinal flora is one of the body's main defences against infection of the intestines, with aggressive interaction between normal flora and invading pathogens.

The prenatal intestinal tract is sterile. In breast-fed babies a stable microflora of mainly *Lactobacillus bifidus* becomes predominant. Bottle-fed or formula-fed babies have intestinal microflora that more closely resembles that of adults, where bacteroides and bifidobacteria are the major groups. In the intestinal tract of very elderly persons, the number of bifido-bacteria decreases significantly.

PART TWO

What are the main causes of digestive problems?

CHAPTER 2

Who is most likely to suffer from digestive problems?

This chapter discusses five inherent factors, i.e. factors that you cannot control, or that you can do little about. But being aware of the impact that these have on the digestive tract may help you to take note of factors relating to diet and lifestyle where you *can* exercise control.

Heredity

Does indigestion 'run in the family'? Some problems of digestive enzyme deficiency, absorption and metabolism may be inherited, to predispose you to certain difficulties; some problems may have been caused by faulty foetal development; some sensitivities are noticeable in childhood; others develop in later years as the activities of cells and muscles decline.

The tendency to have ulcers can run in families. The risk of developing a duodenal or gastric ulcer is three times greater in people who have close relatives with these ailments. Your blood group appears to influence whether you develop ulcers; studies have shown that people with group O blood are at greater risk of having duodenal ulcer disease.

Heredity obviously plays some part in gastrointestinal cancers; for example, the Bonapartes had a great tendency towards cancer of the stomach. The condition known as *familial polyposis* of the colon is inherited, and is a precursor of colon cancer.

Genetic factors are not under our control at present, although future research may pinpoint defective genes and possibly alter them.

Race

Are you black or white? If you are black, you may live in Africa or your ancestors may have come from there, which would predispose you towards indigestion after drinking milk and milk products – lactose intolerance. If you are white, you may have gluten intolerance and find wheat products indigestible – a condition which is rare among blacks. Blacks appear to have a higher incidence of ulcers than whites, including a higher death rate from complications.

Sex

More than twice as many men as women have duodenal ulcers, although incidence among men and women is about equally divided for gastric ulcers. More women than men appear to suffer from inflammatory bowel disease. Women may have digestive upsets due to altered hormonal levels as part of a premenstrual syndrome of change: physical changes, emotional changes such as increased anxiety, and behavioural changes such as unusual food cravings. Many women around the time of their menstrual period experience nausea, heartburn, constipation or diarrhoea triggered by the autonomic nervous system or changing levels of oestrogen and progesterone which affect the contractions of the oesophagus and stomach. Doctors recommend avoiding caffeine, fats, sweets, salt and alcohol during premenstrual days.

Young women taking birth-control pills have an increased incidence of gallstones. Birth-control pills containing large amounts of oestrogen can increase risk of blood clots in vessels supplying the intestine, and cause abdominal pains and bloody diarrhoea (*ischaemic colitis*). Progesterone-containing contraceptive pills can reduce pressure of the lower oesophageal sphincter, which may increase heartburn.

After menopause, women have a decline in digestive secretions, and the action of adrenal glands may trigger occasional diarrhoea, resulting in poor digestion and absorption, or constipation and elimination problems.

Women seem more prone than men to embarking on extreme

slimming diets, using laxatives, diuretics and hazardous medications to take off weight, succeeding in giving themselves watery diarrhoea.

Ageing

Natural laws dictate when human cells will multiply, grow in number and effectiveness, then gradually reduce cell count and activity – and finally disappear. Other factors such as chronic diseases and lifestyle may determine and accelerate the rate at which cells evolve or are maintained.

With each stage in life, nutritional needs vary and your digestive tract undergoes changes. There are natural differences and changes in mucosa, acid secretions, digestive enzymes, cell decline, muscular activity, hormonal activity, and the absorption from foods of nutrients, vitamins and minerals, with the result that the intestine does not function as effectively as it did in earlier years.

Ageing may bring difficulties in chewing because of the loss of natural teeth, and the wearing of dentures; a reduction in taste perception (resulting from a decline in smell receptors) may curb appetite or lead to overuse of salt or sweeteners to enhance food flavours.

There may be a reduced level of acidity in the older stomach, and an altered balance of colonic bacteria. Some elderly persons who are malnourished have an increase in bacterial overgrowth which produces diarrhoea. Many people over the age of 70 suffer hardening of arteries, which can reduce the blood supply to the intestines, and cause *abdominal angina* (abdominal pain that may be difficult to diagnose). Advancing years bring an increased incidence in the development of gallstones, diverticula ('pockets' in the wall of the intestine), colon polyps, cancers of the digestive tract and irritable bowel syndrome. Weakened anal sphincter muscles in the elderly increase the risk of faecal incontinence.

The onset of chronic diseases such as arthritis and vascular diseases that necessitate taking medications regularly can have an effect on the gastrointestinal tract. See the section on chronic diseases in Chapter 4.

Culture

Problems of the gastrointestinal tract are worldwide, of course, but there appears to be a relationship between where you live and the type of problems you may have. Studies of food habits from country to country indicate that differences in food and lifestyle can produce different digestive problems and diseases. In the West, about 30 per cent of cancers are diet-related: the high proportion of fat in the Western diet results in cancers of the colon and rectum; diverticulosis (the presence of many diverticula or pockets in the intestine) is more common in developed Western societies but rare in parts of Africa. On the other hand, the Japanese preference for pickled vegetables is known to lead to cancer of the oesophagus. American Pima Indians have a high incidence of gallstone formation.

CHAPTER 3

How your diet affects the digestive system

The factors in this chapter are related to foods, drinks and diet: how much you eat, the type of diet you have, and the safe handling of food.

Overeating

Too much. Too quickly. Too late. The painful truth is that many common problems of indigestion are caused by simply eating too much food so that your system is overburdened and overwhelmed. Bolting too much food, you go far beyond the time when your brain signals the end of hunger and appetite is satisfied. The perception of taste-buds becomes dulled. Food is improperly chewed before swallowing. The weight of food forces the release of the oesophageal sphincter muscle to relax to cause the start of belching and heartburn. The stomach swells, pressure forces food back up into the oesophagus, and you taste the acid reflux. Large quantities of gastric juices are triggered, pancreatic bicarbonate may be insufficient to cope, causing damage to wall linings. Digestive enzymes are outnumbered by the quantity of food coming down to challenge them. Undigested particles fermented by colon bacteria cause flatulence.

How much food do you really need? Table 2 shows the average number of daily calories for moderately active people.

What you can do
Space meals evenly throughout the day, preferably in the earlier hours. Eating one heavy meal a day, dumping too much food on your system all at once, is asking for trouble; having a heavy meal and then going straight to bed is a digestive disaster. Three

TABLE 2
CALORIES AND DIETARY FAT

Total daily calories	Recommended for:	Recommended calories from fat (30%)	Grams of fat
1400	Women 45+	420	47
1600	Women 18–44	480	53
1800	Girls 12–17	540	60
2000	Children 6–11 and men 55+	600	67
2400	Men 18–54	720	80
2600	Boys 12–17	780	87

evenly-spaced meals are better. Some dietitians recommend six mini-meals throughout the day, because each time you eat you 'rev up' the metabolism mechanism; in this way you may assist weight control and avoid wild peaks and valleys in levels of blood sugars and fats (lipids).

What makes you overeat? Is it the habit in your family to have large meals? Do you link big portions with bulging muscles, body-building and athletic prowess? Or are you a gourmet who enjoys multi-course meals? Do you love to cook, and find yourself preparing far more food than you and your family really need? Do you hate to see food go to waste and eat leftovers from other plates? Are you a company executive who has to attend heavy business dinners or a politician who must go to official banquets? Do you enjoy entertaining? Is your idea of a good time making everyone eat too much? Or do you overeat as a means of comfort when feeling stressed, anxious or angry?

Bulimia

Overeating is also part of the gorge/purge syndrome known as *bulimia nervosa*. This eating disorder is largely psychological and emotional. Bulimic behaviour is defined as recurrent episodes of rapid consumption of large amounts of food in a short period, followed by self-induced vomiting, often using syrup of ipecacuanha, laxative use, rigorous dieting or fasting to counteract gorging.

A bulimic can have teeth rotting and decaying rapidly with the bile acids from frequent vomiting, inflammation of the oesophagus, and heartburn as the oesophageal sphincter is weakened. A bulimic risks kidney failure and liver damage. Overuse of harsh laxatives can result in impaired muscle tone and loss of normal bowel function. Food nutrients have little chance of being absorbed, leading to malnutrition.

Another eating disorder related to bulimia is *anorexia nervosa*, which is dieting to the point of starvation, with an obsessive desire to be ultra-thin. Appetite is lost. Although limiting the amount of food one eats is a normal way of trying to lose weight, it is not normal to stop eating to the point of emaciation.

What you can do
Seek the help of a doctor, therapist or nutritionist for counselling. Write to the address in the Resources section for further information.

The wrong type of food

Too much fat

Look again at Table 2. Nutritionists recommend that the percentage of fat in the diet should be no more than one-third, preferably less, and not eaten all at one meal. Fatty foods
- stimulate acid secretion.
- induce a weakening of the lower oesophageal sphincter to allow reflux of stomach contents to cause heartburn.
- can be broken down by gut bacteria into substances that can initiate cancers of the colon and rectum.
- increase the production of bile acids.
- may trigger cancer of the liver, with a constant overload of unused fatty acids.
- possibly induce cancer of the pancreas.
- are metabolized easily to body fat stores, encouraging obesity.
- when undigested in the intestine, actually grease it, causing diarrhoea.

What you can do

Avoid deep-fried, batter-coated, greasy dishes, chips or French fries, whole milk, high-fat cheeses, rich cream sauces, sardines packed in oil, and fatty potato crisps. Many commercial ready-prepared processed foods are fat-laden, but the fat is concealed; home cooking puts you in control. Go for skimmed milk, nonfat dairy products, well-trimmed lean meat and skinless poultry.

Too little fibre

A diet lacking fibre needs less saliva, and thus deprives the stomach of saliva's acid-buffering action. Low-fibre foods require less chewing than fibrous ones. Insufficient fibre allows food to spend too long in your digestive tract. Conditions are created for diverticulosis, diverticulitis, constipation, appendicitis, Crohn's disease, colon polyps, cancer of the colon, and painful problems of the anus such as fissures and haemorrhoids.

Dietary fibre (or roughage or bulk) is the portion of plants which is not broken down by chemical action in the digestive system. The fibrous parts of meat are not considered dietary fibre, and there is no fibre in dairy products. Fibre is found in fruits, vegetables, whole grains and legumes (dried beans and peas).

Table 3 gives examples of the amounts of fibre in some common foods, the calories per serving and the calorie/fibre ratio (the lower the number, the better).

What you can do

Most people can benefit by having between 25 and 35g of dietary fibre each day; not more than 35g daily because of possible harmful effects such as diarrhoea and deficiencies of iron, calcium and copper.

Doctors and dietitians warn against too sudden a change in the diet. It takes time for the gastrointestinal (GI) tract to adapt. It is important to increase intake of dietary fibre *gradually* to accustom your tract to increased contractions, and thus avoid cramping and unwanted diarrhoea. Bran should never be eaten dry, because it can clog the digestive system. Drink plenty of liquids (water is ideal) to avoid impaction of solids. Have at least four to six glasses a day: a glass first thing in the morning, and 15 minutes before meals.

TABLE 3

EXAMPLES OF FIBRE AND CALORIE CONTENT OF FOODS

Food	Serving size	Fibre/ serving (grams)	Calories/ serving	Cal./ Fibre ratio
Cereals:				
All-Bran	⅓ cup/1oz/30g	8.5	71	8.4
Bran Buds	⅓ cup/1oz/30g	7.9	73	9.2
Bran Flakes	¾ cup/1oz/30g	4.0	93	23.2
Fruits:				
Apple with skin	1 apple	4.3	81	18.8
Banana	1 banana	1.6	105	65.6
Peach	1 peach	0.6	37	61.7
Pear with skin	1 pear	4.1	98	23.9
Raspberries	1 cup/4oz/115g	5.8	61	10.5
Pulses/legumes, cooked:				
Baked beans	½ cup/3oz/85g	3.3	118	35.8
Kidney beans	½ cup/3oz/85g	3.2	112	35.0
Lentils	½ cup/3oz/85g	4.0	115	28.7
Haricot/Navy beans	½ cup/3oz/85g	3.3	129	39.1
Borlotti/Pinto beans	½ cup/3oz/85g	3.4	117	34.4
Mixed dishes:				
Beef and bean chilli	1 cup/9oz/255g	1.7	374	220.0
Lettuce salad (no dressing)	1 cup/2oz/60g	0.4	10	25.0
Pancakes, wholemeal	2 pancakes	1.8	250	138.9
Split pea soup	¾ cup/6 fl oz	5.9	172	29.1
Tuna sandwich on wholemeal bread	1 sandwich	2.8	305	108.9
Vegetables, cooked:				
Brussels sprouts	½ cup/2½oz/75g	2.5	33	13.2
Carrots	½ cup/2½oz/75g	1.5	35	23.3
Green peas	½ cup/3oz/85g	3.0	67	22.3
Potato, baked, with skin	1 potato/7oz/200g	1.3	220	169.2
Spinach, frozen	½ cup/3oz/90g	3.0	27	9.0
Courgettes/ Zucchini	½ cup/3oz/90g	0.4	14	35.0

Spices and flavourings

Many people have trouble with food ingredients such as hot peppers, chilli powder, cumin, nutmeg, ginger, cinnamon, all-spice, spearmint and peppermint. Also citrus fruits and juices, tomatoes and tomato products, garlic, onions and green cabbage.

What you can do
Obviously you need to avoid whatever you find troublesome.

Effervescent drinks

When bubbles are naturally present in beverages, or added during processing or mixing, they will add to the gases in your stomach, increase distention, weaken the lower oesophageal sphincter to create heartburn and belching, cause cramping, and increase flatulence. Gas can collect anywhere in the colon.

What you can do
Avoid trouble-makers such as sparkling mineral waters, sparkling wines and champagnes, gassy beers, carbonated mixers and fizzy soft drinks. Even air introduced into whipped cream, frothy omelettes and popcorn can sometimes create intestinal gas.

Caffeine

Caffeine may be your enemy. Caffeine is a drug. It is found in coffee beans, tea leaves, cacao beans (from which cocoa is made) and cola nuts (the source of cola flavouring used in many soft drinks). It belongs to a class of chemical compounds known as methylxanthines, which are found naturally in more than sixty plant species.

Caffeine is in coffee (regular, decaffeinated and acid-neutralized), tea, chocolates, drinking chocolate, cocoa, baked goods, frozen dairy products, gelatines, puddings and confectionery, some herbal teas and many soft drinks.

The amount of caffeine in a cup of coffee or tea depends on your personal taste and preference; you may like coffee or tea strong or weak. Caffeine content is influenced by the variety of bean or leaf, where it was grown, particle size (coffee grind or tea-leaf cut), and the method of brewing or steeping.

Caffeine is an ingredient in more than 1,000 non-prescription drug products as well as numerous prescription drugs. Most often it is used in weight control remedies, alertness or stay-awake tablets, headache and pain relief remedies, allergy medicines, cold products and diuretics (urine-inducing medicine). Caffeine may be part of prescriptions for migraine headaches, tension headaches and muscle relaxants. It is possible that people over 50 who need several medications may have more caffeine from drug sources than from their diet. Caffeine can cause

- decrease of appetite.
- inflammation of the oesophagus.
- heartburn, with the relaxation and weakening of the lower oesophageal sphincter to allow reflux of the contents of the stomach.
- stimulation of acid secretion, producing inflammation of the stomach and duodenum.
- ulcers. Most studies show that caffeine does not *cause* ulcers, but may exacerbate pre-existing conditions and increase symptoms. Caffeine is harmful and painful to both gastric and duodenal ulcers, especially when taken on an empty stomach.
- diarrhoea, due to irritation of the colon.
- possibly cancer of the pancreas, colon and rectum.
- increase in jitteriness and symptoms of stress.

What you can do
Read food labels before buying. Stop consuming everything known to contain caffeine: coffee, tea, chocolate, and caffeine-labelled soft drinks. Decaffeinated coffees and teas are not entirely caffeine-free, and some studies have cast doubt about their safety if drunk in considerable quantities. Limit consumption of decaffeinated coffees and teas to no more than one or two cups per day. If labels on medicine are unclear, ask your chemist, pharmacist or doctor.

Alternatives to caffeine-containing drinks can be hot water with a squeeze of lemon juice, bouillon made from meat or vegetable extracts, miso broth, soya milk, commercial herb tea (read the label to be sure it is caffeine-free), or grain-based beverages such as Aromalt, Barleycup, Caro, and Prewett's Instant Chicory (or Caffix, Postum, and Pero in the USA).

Food allergies and food intolerance

Many people have physical reactions after eating certain foods – allergies, sensitivity or an intolerance.

Allergies

A true food *allergy* or sensitivity involves the body's immune system. Allergic reactions to foods may include not only stomach cramps, diarrhoea, vomiting, but *also* asthma and sneezing, hives or skin rash and other symptoms. Reactions may occur immediately, or hours after eating. The chief offenders among food allergens are cow's milk, chocolate and cola, corn, eggs or egg whites, cereal grains (wheat, rice, barley, oats, wild rice, millet and rye). Other food allergens include pork, beef, fish, shellfish, onion, garlic, banana and some nuts.

If you suspect one particular food, stop eating it for three weeks. If symptoms subside, you can gradually reintroduce the food item to see if symptoms return. Milk protein allergy is an uncommon sensitivity generally found in bottle-fed newborn babies, but it usually disappears before the age of four.

Food intolerance

Intolerance, on the other hand, is caused by an enzyme deficiency, a toxin, or a disease. Food intolerance can cause symptoms similar to food allergies: stomach cramping and diarrhoea, bloating and wind, but *not* usually the asthma-like symptoms. Lactose and gluten are two items that many people do not tolerate well.

Lactose intolerance

Many people say that 'milk doesn't agree with them' and are unable to drink milk or consume other dairy products without suffering cramps, bloating and intestinal gas.

Lactose intolerance pertains to the natural sugars in milk, a combination of glucose and galactose called *lactose*. The enzyme lactase in your intestinal tract is necessary to split these milk-sugars for absorption through the intestinal wall. A shortage of lactase can give many people trouble in comfortably digesting large quantities of milk or milk products, because much of the undigested milk-sugar stays in the intestines, with the natural gut bacteria growing on it and producing wind. You can suffer nausea, stomach ache, diarrhoea and bloating for up to 10 to 12 hours.

Three different types of lactase deficiency are known:

1. **Congenital** lactase deficiency, which is very rare, in which babies are born with limited or no ability to produce lactase, so all lactose-containing foods must be eliminated from the diet.
2. **Temporary** lactase deficiency, due to stomach surgery, certain drugs (such as anti-inflammatory medicines for arthritis and some antibiotics), or radiation treatment in the area of the abdomen. If damaged tissue in the lining of the small intestine subsequently recovers to promote growth of healthy lactase-producing cells, lactose tolerance should return to normal.
3. **Inherited** lactase deficiency, which affects millions of people. This most common type is caused by a gradual decrease in lactase production after the age of two years. Certain ethnic groups show a definite decline in lactase with age, although lactase production during infancy and early childhood is usually adequate. Officially, lactose intolerance in the UK has only been noted as a problem for people of African origin, with an estimated incidence of about 1 per cent of the total population. Table 4 shows the estimated prevalence of lactase deficiency in healthy adults in different population groups around the world.

So far, no method has been found to restore general lactase levels in the intestines. But lactose intolerance is not like an allergy, where the reaction is unrelated to dose.

What you can do
The best approach is to determine your own personal level of tolerance to milk. Usually you can overcome the problem if you

- drink small amounts of milk throughout the day.
- combine milk with other foods.

TABLE 4

PERCENTAGE OF PEOPLES WITH
LACTASE DEFICIENCY

Group	Percentage with lactase deficiency
American blacks	70
American whites	8
Arabs	78
Bantus	90
Danes	2
Filipinos	90
Finns	18
Greek Cypriots	85
Greenland Eskimos	80
Indians	50
Israelis	58
Japanese	85
Peruvians	70
Swiss	7
Taiwanese	85
Thais	90

- serve milk at room temperature or slightly warmed.
- buy lactose-reduced milk and cottage cheese.
- take milk-digestant tablets containing lactase just prior to eating a lactose-containing food.
- treat milk with lactase enzyme products such as 'LactAid', widely available as drops or tablets.
- choose fermented milk products such as buttermilk, sour cream and yogurt, because the fermentation process uses up some of the lactose. People in countries where there is high lactase deficiency usually eat yogurt and other cultured milks.
- buy cured cheeses such as natural Cheddar, Gouda and Edam which are usually more digestible, because much of the lactose is lost during production.

Gluten intolerance

Gluten is in fact a generic term for two other proteins, prolamine and glutalin, which occur in varying amounts in different grains. Gluten intolerance occurs when these combinations of proteins – found in wheat, rye, oats, barley and buckwheat – irritate the lining of the small intestine. An underlying cause maybe a deficiency in peptidase enzymes necessary for digestion of gluten. As a result, nutrients are inadequately absorbed from the intestine, and malnutrition can develop if the problem is left untreated. Gluten intolerance can range from mild to severe: diarrhoea, and fatty foul-smelling stools, poor appetite and abnormal growth – the symptoms of coeliac disease, which is concerned with the malabsorption of fat. Coeliac disease, which is probably an inherited defect, was formerly called non-tropical sprue. In infants, onset usually occurs gradually, causing intestinal upsets during the first year of life and becoming fully developed during the second year. Most children improve in adolescence and adulthood, but the disease may recur. Adult coeliac disease commonly begins after the age of 30 years, creating constipation alternating with diarrhoea. Coeliac disease is almost exclusively found in white children, uncommon in blacks, and never found in Orientals.

Eliminating certain cereal grains provides dramatic relief of symptoms. Some coeliacs may or may not tolerate the gluten in rye, oats, barley and buckwheat, but most have an allergy to wheat. They generally need to omit from their diet wheat flour, wheat starch, and combinations of flours that include wheat. Oats have only about one-quarter to one-fifth the gluten-type proteins that wheat has. Buckwheat is often confused with wheat, but it is a member of another plant family; however, some people are also sensitive to buckwheat. Some experts believe that small amounts of gluten can cause damage to the intestines of a person with coeliac sprue. The proteins in corn, rice, soya bean and tapioca flours, and potato, arrowroot and cornflours contain no problem gluten.

What you can do

Avoid problems of food sensitivity or intolerance by being a label reader. Food ingredients made from milk, eggs, corn or wheat are sometimes listed on the label only by their technical names, so here are the words to look for:

Milk: caseinate, casein, curds, dry milk solids, nonfat dry milk, and whey.

Eggs: albumin, ovomucin, ovomucoid, vitellin, ovovitellin, livetin, powdered or dried egg, ovoglobulin.

Wheat: bran, plain flour, self-raising flour, wheat flour, farina, graham flour, malt, wheat germ, wholewheat flour, and wheat starch.

Gluten: includes all items listed under wheat, plus barley, oats, rye and buckwheat.

Corn: dextrose, deximaltose, corn syrup, corn sugar, corn oil, corn alcohol, cornflour, and glucose.

Vitamin and mineral supplements

The Recommended Dietary Allowances (RDA) for each vitamin and mineral are not minimum amounts. They include an extra margin to cover wide variations in needs. Digestive problems can be traced to overdoses of supplementary vitamins and minerals, or to certain deficiencies. For instance

An overdose of:	may cause:
Vitamin A	nausea, diarrhoea, liver damage.
Nicotinic acid (a form of the B vitamin niacin)	irritated stomach lining, peptic ulcers, diabetes.
Vitamin C	nausea, vomiting, diarrhoea, kidney stones.
Vitamin E	liver dysfunction.
Vitamin K	jaundice.
Calcium	nausea, vomiting, constipation.
Potassium	stomach ulceration.
Iron	liver damage, blackened stools.
Sodium	vomiting, diarrhoea.
Zinc	nausea, diarrhoea.

A deficiency of:	may cause:
Chloride	vomiting, diarrhoea.

Potassium.....................vomiting, diarrhoea.
Sodium........................vomiting.

What you can do
All vitamins and supplements should be kept locked away from children. Five iron pills can be fatal to a three-year-old.

Unsafe food

'It must have been something I ate.'

Primitive humans sought to satisfy hunger by trying out seeds, mushrooms, insects, toads, shellfish, and practically anything that grew, flew, crawled or swam. Many of our ancient ancestors must have been assaulted with poisonous plants, contaminated foods, deadly moulds and bacteria, and millions died annually because of foul food and water.

Food can become contaminated in a variety of ways. Some organisms cause food to spoil, rot or turn bad. That's a help because you know you have to throw it away. However, it is often impossible to tell what is contaminated, as some food may smell, look and taste perfectly good; it may be several hours after eating contaminated food before poisoning becomes evident. You don't deliberately swallow poison, but accidentally eating toxic food can be just as dangerous.

Gastrointestinal symptoms include nausea, vomiting and diarrhoea – a cluster of problems sometimes known as 'gastroenteritis'. Illness can vary in intensity. It may be so mild that you barely notice it, or you pass it off as an upset stomach. On the other hand, serious food poisoning might result in a lengthy hospital stay and in some cases can be fatal. Especially vulnerable are newborn babies, children, pregnant mothers, the elderly or those who have a high risk of infection (such as cancer and AIDS patients, and persons taking certain antibiotics).

In general, toxicity is dose-related: the smaller the dose, the smaller the effect. Your body can usually handle small amounts, but when you overwhelm the natural defence mechanisms by taking in too much at one time, or too much too often, you get into trouble.

What you can do

Key points in avoiding food poisoning are 1) handling food extremely carefully, and 2) eating a variety of foods, to spread out the risk. To lessen your chances of food poisoning:

- Wash your hands after using the toilet, and every time you handle food.
- Don't buy eggs that are soiled or cracked as they can contain harmful bacteria. Refrigerate eggs and use within a week. Eggs should be fully cooked.
- Don't drink raw unpasteurized milk.
- If mould develops on cheeses (other than mould that is an intrinsic part of cheese such as Stilton and veined Cheshire) throw them away.
- Moulds on foods with a high sugar content, such as jams and jellies, may be contaminated with *Aspergillus glaucus*. Discard the jars.
- Check breads, cereals, nuts and seeds for moulds. Discard contaminated foods.
- Refrigerate meats and poultry and use in a day or two, otherwise freeze them. Thaw foods in the refrigerator, not on the countertop. Never eat raw or rare beefburgers.
- Check ham labels for cooking instructions. Fresh ham, like other fresh pork, must be cooked to 80 degrees C (170 degrees F).
- Stuff poultry just before cooking, not the day before. Remove stuffing promptly from the cooked bird and serve separately.
- Buy fish and shellfish from reputable markets. Don't eat raw shellfish, raw or lightly-marinated fish dishes such as ceviche, sushi and sashimi. Eat several varieties of fish species, to minimize your intake of fish that may be contaminated. Clean seafood thoroughly, and keep refrigerated.
- Don't eat green potatoes, or bad potatoes. Thoroughly remove potato 'eyes': toxic solanine glyco-alkaloids are concentrated in these spots.
- Never taste wild mushrooms without first getting expert opinion on identification. It is crucial to recognize differences in mushroom size, shape, colour, texture, habitat and smell. All edible wild mushrooms should be cooked; some species when eaten raw are known to produce digestive upsets.

- To avoid potential residues of pesticides, wash all produce. Peel produce when possible or appropriate. Discard celery tops and outer stalks, and outer leaves of cabbage and lettuce. Avoid waxed fruits.
- Never eat rhubarb leaves; these contain anthraquine glycosides, soluble oxalates which can cause kidney damage.
- Never eat the seeds of apples, pears, peaches, apricots, plums and citrus fruits. Cyanide poisoning can result from eating quantities of seeds. Warn the children.
- Buy herbal teas produced only by reputable manufacturers and sold by dealers you can trust. Herbal teas should only be taken in moderation – no more than two cups a day. Never collect and experiment with wild herbs. Death can result because of confusing and consuming one wild plant for another. All self-treatment with herbs is potentially hazardous.
- Warn the children against eating any part of ornamental garden plants.
- Never buy crushed or dented tinned foods. Use cans within one or two years of purchase. Tinned foods stored in high temperatures can spoil; temperatures below 25°C (75°F) are best. If tins freeze because of storage in sub-zero conditions (in a basement or left in the car), check for swollen cans which may be hazardous.
- Know the warning signs of botulism: leaking, bulging or badly dented tins; cracked jars or jars with loose or bulging lids; seepage or mould around seals; canned food with a bad or musty odour; any container that spurts liquid when you open it, small bubbles in the contents, or cloudy liquid. DON'T EVEN TRY TO TASTE A TINY DROP!
- If you do your own canning and preserving, be sure you are using the newest techniques; some older methods are now considered unsafe. Only preserve good quality, undamaged fruit.

There is more about food poisoning and parasites in Chapter 10.

CHAPTER 4

How your lifestyle affects the digestive system

The factors in this chapter are broadly related to lifestyles – what you do, your personal habits, how you react to your surroundings and environment, and other influences.

Alcohol

Alcohol is a drug. For many people it's practically a social obligation in order to have fun. But it can be dangerous. In fact, a common word for drunkenness, 'intoxication', comes from the Greek *toxikon* meaning 'arrow poison'. So it can be said that by using alcohol carelessly, you risk shooting yourself in several vital organs at once.

It is the amount of alcohol you drink that counts and not the particular kind of drink that the alcohol is in. The percentage of alcohol in drinks is half of its proof: 80 proof vodka, gin, whisky or brandy contains 40 per cent alcohol; a beer that is 8 proof is 4 per cent alcohol. Fortified wines, such as port, Madeira and sherry have about 20 per cent alcohol; table wines have about 10 per cent alcohol. Many medications contain alcohol, such as many cough medicines and remedies for colds and congestion, because alcohol is a better solvent and provides a longer shelf-life than a water solution.

Alcohol has calories, but is not a food that needs to be digested. It goes through the stomach and intestinal wall, straight into your bloodstream. The liver metabolizes 95 per cent of alcohol in the body; the rest leaves the body in saliva, perspiration and breath. If the stomach is empty, the alcohol is rapidly absorbed, but if food is present, it has to wait its turn to come into contact with the walls of the digestive tract, and there is some delay.

If an expectant mother drinks alcohol, so does the foetus, increasing the risk of abnormalities. Breast milk has the same concentration of alcohol as the mother's blood after drinking.

A single enzyme, alcohol dehydrogenase, or ADH, starts the process of breaking down alcohol in the liver, but ADH is limited in quantity, and this limits the rate at which you can assimilate alcohol. ADH is present in the body not for the times you drink alcohol but to digest the alcohol sometimes produced inside the body when metabolizing carbohydrates. With age, the liver becomes less efficient at dealing with alcohol, so tolerance slowly declines.

Apart from increasing your risk of brain damage, heart disease and heart attacks, alcohol can do considerable damage to the gastrointestinal tract, such as

- an upset stomach, which is the result of alcohol's effects either on the brain, or directly on the digestive tract, with irritation of any tissue that it touches. Ethanol in alcohol influences gastrointestinal secretions, motility (movement) and normal patterns of gut bacteria.
- stomach ulcers. Alcohol in the stomach promotes the secretion of large amounts of gastric juice. Beer is a common offender for stimulating stomach-acid secretion, and worsening an existing ulcerous condition.
- disorders of the pancreas.
- mouth and throat cancers. Alcohol promotes the action of carcinogens in tobacco. If you drink heavily and smoke heavily, you have up to 15 times the risk of developing oral cancer than non-drinkers and non-smokers.
- hangover symptoms, which generally include nausea, maybe vomiting and diarrhoea or a change in bowel movements. A hangover can give you a dry mouth, water loss, and a feeling of malaise due to derangement of acid-base balance in your tissues.
- malnutrition, when heavy drinking makes you careless about having regular healthy meals.
- injury to the liver. Every time you drink too much, cells die and are replaced by scar tissue. The scarring hinders the liver's ability to function. Several ailments are included under

the heading 'Alcoholic liver disease': one is fatty liver, marked by the buildup of fat deposits on the liver; alcoholic hepatitis is the result of the liver becoming inflamed and liver cells dying; and the most serious is cirrhosis of the liver, which strikes one in five alcoholics. It is characterized by scarring of the liver tissue serious enough to produce a breakdown of the organ, leaving it unable to function. The disease is irreversible and often fatal.

- Changes in the liver caused by too much alcohol can speed up the metabolism of some drugs, such as anticonvulsants, anticoagulants and diabetes drugs. They become less effective because they do not stay in the body long enough. An alcohol-damaged liver is less able to metabolize or process other drugs, causing them to remain in the system too long. This is particularly serious when the drugs are anti-psychotic (phenothiazines) which can cause further liver damage.
- The carbon dioxide in champagne, effervescent wines and bubbly mixed drinks, and the gassiness in beers, can induce the opening of sphincter valves, thus increasing belching, reflux and flatulence.
- Over-drinking can increase the drawing in of breath and the risk of choking on your own vomit. Under the influence of alcohol, the body's reflexes to cough and vomit do not work correctly, so you have a greater chance that something lodged in your trachea will choke you to death.

The worst thing for a hangover is aspirin, which can cause internal bleeding and further damage the lining of digestive tissues. Having a nip of 'the hair of the dog that bit you', i.e. whatever you were drinking the night before, will only prolong the agony. The cure for a hangover is *time* for your body to recover from the big shock it has received.

What you can do
If you have a drinking problem, the best choice is Alcoholics Anonymous. Look in your telephone directory, or write to the address given in the Resources section at the back of this guide.

What the doctor can do
For control of alcohol consumption, a physician will sometimes

prescribe disulfiram ('Antabuse' by C.P. Pharmaceuticals) which is formulated to cause palpitations, flushing, sweating, shortness of breath or dizziness when even a small amount of drink is taken or other drugs containing alcohol are consumed.

Smoking

Cigarettes put physical stress on the body. Apart from the other ravages caused by tobacco such as lung cancer, respiratory problems and heart disease, smoking has considerable impact on digestion.

- Smoking and nicotine reduce the efficiency of taste-buds, reduce appetite and affect the secretion of saliva.
- Smoking induces heartburn (oesophageal reflux).
- It can increase the motility (movement) of the colon, and make a spastic colon worse.
- It can reduce the efficiency of caloric storage as the body has difficulty in extracting the maximum nutrients from food.
- Nicotine affects hormonal balance so that messenger hormones cannot function properly. Pancreatic fluid secretion and bicarbonate may become inhibited, predisposing a smoker to develop duodenal and possibly gastric ulcers.
- Smoking is associated with the incidence, slow healing, relapse and increased mortality from ulcerous disease. Stopping smoking promotes healing of gastric ulcers.
- Tobacco is responsible for many different types of cancer in the GI tract, including cancers of the mouth, pharynx, oesophagus, stomach, pancreas and liver. In the Western world, cancer of the oesophagus appears to be associated with population groups who smoke cigarettes and are heavy drinkers. Smokers develop pancreatic cancer 10 to 15 years sooner than non-smokers.
- Smoking significantly alters the effect of certain drugs such as pentazocine and theophylline on the function of the liver.
- Heavy smokers who are also heavy drinkers often suffer oxygen deficiency (hypoxia), which can accelerate the progression of alcoholic liver disease.
- Nicotine and motherhood do not mix. Apart from inducing

birth defects, nicotine can result in a lower birth-weight baby, and reduce the flow of a mother's milk. Nicotine can be passed on to the baby through breast milk and lead to jitteriness in the baby.

Tobacco consumption can take different forms: cigarettes, pipe tobacco, cigars, chewing tobacco, snuff (usually sniffed up the nostrils or sometimes chewed), and clove cigarettes (which contain 60 per cent tobacco). In some countries, such as India, the people use pan (betel, chewed with slaked lime), bidi (or biri) – a cheap home-grown tobacco wrapped in leaves, and hookah (or hukka) – a pipe with smoke passing through water. All these forms and methods have different tar and nicotine contents, and consequently varying effects on the GI tract.

Chewing tobacco and snuff have a direct relationship with the development of cancer of the gums and mouth. Smokeless tobacco can cause gums to recede, make teeth vulnerable to falling out, discolour teeth, increase tooth sensitivity, and produce slow-healing cuts and sores in the mouth.

According to a report from the Office of Population Censuses and Surveys, 34 per cent of people in Britain are smokers, and of this number, 32 per cent are women. Furthermore, women were smoking more cigarettes per week in 1984 than in 1972. By the age of sixteen, 25 per cent of girls were smoking compared with 16 per cent of boys. Medical authorities consider the age at which you start to smoke is crucial, because the earlier you begin, the longer is your exposure to tobacco and the risk of smoking-related illnesses and diseases.

What you can do
The time to quit is NOW! Join a group in a cigarette withdrawal clinic, or contact addresses in the Resources section for counsel and self-help pamphlets.

You can fight nicotine addiction with various products available at chemists and drug stores: smoking-deterrent chewing gum, a variety of filters to be attached to cigarettes, reducing tar and nicotine inhaled, or tablets such as 'Test 60' and 'Nicobrevin'.

Street drugs and drug abuse

Apart from the mind-bending and mind-scrambling produced by street drugs, these substances and their impurities can have long-term complications on the functioning of the digestive system.

The sniffing of glues and aerosols (aeroplane glue, plastic cements, paints, lacquers, thinners, cleaning fluids, petrol, lighter fuel) can damage the liver and kidneys.

Amphetamines ('uppers') and methamphetamines ('crank' and 'speed') create loss of appetite down to starvation levels, leading to malnutrition. People who inject amphetamines risk hepatitis and damage to kidneys. Barbiturates can cause an impairment of liver function, change metabolism, producing deficiencies of hormones and vitamins.

Marijuana's main psychoactive ingredient is Delta-9-tetra-hydrocannabinol (THC) which accumulates and causes damage in the body's fatty tissue such as the liver. Smoking five marijuana cigarettes is the equivalent of smoking 112 tobacco cigarettes.

Cocaine or 'crack' kills the appetite, causes nausea and vomiting; and many habitual users suffer from malnutrition, protein, vitamin and mineral deficiencies, and significant weight loss. Long-term use may damage the liver. Other symptoms include belching, the urge to defecate, and a slowdown of digestion.

Not all drugs are illegally obtained; for instance, many women acquire diet pills with doctors' prescriptions, perhaps without realizing they are becoming increasingly dependent on them.

Drug dependents eventually pay in terms of health, although not every drug abuser pays the same price for the same excess. Among heavy drug users, malnutrition is often the result of erratic and irregular meals, and the function of the liver is impaired, reducing the effectiveness to activate vitamin D.

What you can do
With the right help, drug habits can be broken, though it may take months. Your local health authorities have information about nearby help, drug abuse services and programmes. Or refer to the addresses shown in the Resources section.

Stress

Physical stress

You may be physically stressed, fatigued, overtired after work, a workout at the health centre, or a hard game of tennis. Rest a short while before taking a meal, then eat lightly.

Emotional stress

Anxiety is natural, but it can get out of hand and you can be your own worst enemy. Your mood and psychological state can have a profound impact on the digestive system and cause stomach upsets. You may be worrying because you have an illness, disease or injury, or – more likely – you are feeling strain at the death of a close relative, family problems, money, noisy neighbours, a new job, unbearable workloads or overtime, chronic frustration with tyrannical supervisors, unemployment, retirement, driving in rush-hour traffic. Anger, anxiety, grief, loneliness, interrruptions, noise, speed, and all the threats that life throws at you. It's not the events themselves, but your body's response to stressful conditions which can be a series of physical and chemical changes in your ability to function. But we're all different. What you perceive to be pleasantly stimulating and exciting may cause painful distress to another person.

Stress can

- alter levels of hormones that send signals for digestion.
- suppress appetite.
- cause mouth dryness.
- cause insufficient chewing.
- change the bacterial level in your mouth, resulting in a greater tendency to have teeth decay and loosen.
- close the oesophagus, making it difficult to swallow, creating 'a lump in the throat'.
- weaken the lower oesophageal sphincter, to allow reflux of stomach acid and cause heartburn.
- increase or decrease secretion of stomach acid.
- change enzyme levels that aid digestion.
- cause changes in gastric mucosa.
- create conditions conducive to the formation of ulcers.

- cause the liver to dump cholesterol into the bloodstream.
- alter blood sugar levels to increase any tendency to diabetes.
- increase or decrease peristaltic contractions, to trigger diarrhoea or constipation.
- increase the production of gas.
- cause changes in metabolism to accelerate weight loss or gain.

Most common among young children, especially when first starting school, are symptoms of stomach aches. They are rarely actually ill, but when a stomach ache develops after breakfast, the child is allowed to stay home. These are worried children with a school phobia.

What you can do
A turning point in digestive problems may be when you recognize that stress is your enemy, but how do you cope? There is no single strategy that is best for everyone. See box for suggestions on combating stress.

- Exercise. Do something energetic instead of giving way to anger or bottling it up. Take a walk, play a friendly game of tennis, or do gardening. Deep breathing helps to relieve tension.
- Take time to relax. Ask your family to give you 20 minutes of personal quiet time when you arrive home from work and before you tackle domestic chores. Take short naps. Try meditation. Read a book, do a jigsaw puzzle, listen to beautiful music.
- Develop new interests, new hobbies, to help you forget daily problems: play a musical instrument, take up fishing. Have a pet you can play with and love.
- Have a good cry now and then, as a healthy release of tension.
- Seek advice, forgiveness, or an apology. Discuss problems with a friend you can trust, a counsellor or your clergyman.
- Know your limits. Take a slower approach to life, if you are struggling to fit too many activities into your day, with family responsibilities, work, church and school.
- Stop doing everything yourself, and delegate.

- Don't be a perfectionist.
- Realize that you cannot be so ambitious. Perhaps you can change jobs.
- List priorities – do one thing at a time and postpone the rest.
- Learn to say no. You may be one of those people who too often says yes to requests for time from family and friends, and end up with no time for yourself.
- Get enough rest and eat sensibly. If you are irritable and tense from lack of sleep, or if you are not eating properly, you will be less able to deal with stressful situations.
- Have a really good laugh. Healthy people are said to laugh over 100 times a day. Laughter *is* the world's best medicine.

Exercise

Whether you exercise regularly or are a 'couch potato' can be reflected in the state of your gastrointestinal tract. A reasonable amount of exercise is necessary for the efficient maintenance of all the body's functions. If you are bedridden or confined to a wheelchair you may have sluggish bowels and the weakness that results from muscular inactivity. Elderly people, even if ambulatory, seldom exercise as much as they should, and consequently suffer more problems of constipation and haemorrhoids.

What you can do
Exercise makes an important contribution to good digestion. How much you can manage is up to you. It can be dangerous to embark suddenly on too vigorous a programme if you are unaccustomed to exercise, if you are overweight, or have any kind of cardiac or respiratory ailment. Check with your doctor before beginning any unusual exertion.

Walking is good for almost everyone. It can tone your muscles, perk up the appetite, be a tonic to the digestive system, and give you an overall sense of well-being. You don't have to train for the Olympics or run a marathon every day to gain benefits. Just a couple of 15-minute brisk walks every day are helpful. A walk that doesn't even make you perspire can improve fitness. Light gardening (rhythmic raking of leaves, sweeping paths and pushing the lawn mower) can also get you moving.

Exercise can help too with the control of fats and cholesterol in the blood, help stabilize glucose levels in Type II (non-insulin dependent/maturity onset) diabetics, and assist in weight control. Exercise releases tensions, calms your nerves, helps give you a different outlook on life. But avoid any vigorous aerobics or bending over to weed in the garden just after a meal, which would trigger heartburn. Make exercise a regular habit for life, and do what you enjoy so it doesn't become a bore.

Overweight and obesity

You may weigh several pounds more than you should, and find your indigestion getting worse. Your overweight may be because you are eating more, exercising less, or both. You may be getting less exercise because of a temporary or permanent disability, injury or stroke; or eating more to calm anxiety. Being obese may 'run in the family', or be due to glandular problems. You may like to eat foods that are fatty and have an unbalanced diet. You may have 'gastronomic obesity', if you love to prepare elaborate meals and consider yourself a gourmet. You could be a kitchen food-disposer, nibbling all day long, always cooking, or eating leftovers. Or you could be in a position of authority, and believe it is an advantage to have extra pounds to give you dignity or add weight to your opinions. Whatever the underlying reasons for being overweight, the extra pounds have an impact on your digestion:

- heartburn. Obesity increases pressures within the abdomen, weakening the lower oesophageal sphincter and causing stomach acids to flow back into the oesophagus.
- a greater tendency to have diabetes.
- a higher cholesterol level.
- gallstones, which are generally triggered by a greater production of cholesterol in the liver, resulting in elevated cholesterol levels in the body from a supersaturated bile.

Overall, the risk is about twice that of normal-weight people, and particularly prevalent among obese women.

- an increased risk of cancers of the pancreas and gallbladder (in women) and cancers of the colon and rectum (in men).
- development of haemorrhoids, due to weight or pressure on the vein system.

What you can do
If you need help in loosing weight sensibly, join a local class or Y.M.C.A. group. Or refer to the addresses in the Resources section for information and services.

Pregnancy

Being pregnant and feeding your own baby may bring joy to your heart – but heartburn to your digestive system.

Childbearing causes many chemical as well as physical changes, including alterations in hormone levels and variations in the way your body absorbs nutrients from food. Your food requirements change, you eat more, you may have strange food cravings. As breasts increase in size, they put pressure on oesophagus and stomach contents. The doctor advises you to include more milk and dairy products in your diet, and these have a constipating effect; and closer to your delivery date you probably take less exercise.

Digestive tract problems can include

- decay or loss of teeth, if stores of calcium are depleted for foetal bone formation. See *Brittle Bones and the Calcium Crisis* (Thorsons, 1987).
- increased incidence of heartburn. Up to 80 per cent of women complain of heartburn at some time during preganancy, and between 50 and 60 per cent of expectant mothers experience it during the last trimester. The early increase is due to the effect of progesterone relaxing the lower oesophageal sphincter, other hormonal changes that slow down the digestive system, and by the mechanical pressure of the growing foetus against the stomach. As pregnancy advances, the incidence of reflux oesophagitis increases: heartburn is most marked at 36 weeks.

- vomiting (morning sickness) which may be of psychological origin or due to altered hormone levels and physical changes. Although called morning sickness, it can occur at any time of the day.
- hiatal hernia. As the foetus grows, it exerts more pressure, and occupies more abdominal space.
- a possible increase in the formation of gallstones, because of altered activity of the gallbladder and the ability of bile to form stones. The risk of gallstones increases with the number of pregnancies.
- ulcerative colitis, which occurs in about 25 per cent of women, usually during the first three months of pregnancy.
- women with Crohn's disease will experience a recurrence, not during the pregnancy itself, but about 30 per cent notice a return of symptoms during the first three months after delivery.
- constipation, probably due to progesterone hormones that tend to relax the muscles of the intestines. Late in pregnancy, constipation may be caused by the growing foetus pressing upon the rectum and other organs.
- increase in haemorrhoidal tissue as veins become engorged.

At the same time, women who have ulcers experience dramatic remissions during pregnancy, only to have the disease return perhaps six months after delivery. An active ulcer is practically unknown during pregnancy.

What you can do
To alleviate morning sickness, it is often helpful to eat a small snack of a cracker or dry biscuit before rising in the morning, then remain in bed for about 15 or 20 minutes to allow the mini-meal to settle. Move slowly when you get up. Let plenty of fresh air into the house to remove cooking odours and other household smells that may trigger nausea. If nausea returns during the day, another small snack may do the trick. Gynaecologists often advise eating frequent small meals rather than three normal-sized ones, limiting fats, highly-spiced foods, strong-flavoured vegetables, acidic drinks and citrus juices. Drink liquids *between* rather than with meals.

To avert heartburn, avoid greasy or highly-spiced foods and any others that do not agree with you. Sleep with several pillows to elevate your head. Do *not* take bicarbonate of soda (baking soda) to relieve heartburn, or any other medicines unless your doctor recommends them.

To relieve constipation during pregnancy, there are several things you can do. Drink six to eight glasses of liquids each day. A glass of cold water or juice before breakfast is often effective. Eat fibrous foods such as wholegrain cereals and breads, and raw unpeeled fruits and vegetables. Take some exercise every day. Do not take enemas, laxatives or home remedies unless advised by your doctor.

To prevent haemorrhoids, avoid becoming constipated and don't strain at bowel movements. Lying on your side with your hips on a pillow may relieve haemorrhoids. Or you may get relief from an ice-bag or a compress of clean fabric soaked in cold witch hazel or a solution of Epsom salts. If haemorrhoids bleed, tell your doctor. The problem usually goes away after delivery.

Chronic diseases, their drugs and side effects

In serious illnesses such as diabetes, hepatitis, tuberculosis, certain thyroid disorders and some types of cancer, loss of appetite can be a complication. Drugs needed after cancer surgery often cause mouth sores, nausea, vomiting and diarrhoea. Drugs for chronic conditions can produce prolonged vomiting or bleeding. Some prescription pain pills may increase the risk of such critical problems as peptic ulcers and intestinal perforation. These are warning signals that the drug is causing problems, and you should consult your doctor immediately.

Simple aspirin, or one of the many compounds containing aspirin or salicylic acid, can cause gastritis and increase the risk of gastric ulcers when the painkiller is taken frequently.

When you take antibiotics to combat infections in any part of your body, these medications can kill the normal bacteria in the intestines as well, and allow certain resistant bacteria types to take over the territory usually occupied by the friendly germs. The most frequently recognized, *C. difficile*, produces a poison that can damage the cells that line the colon, resulting in diarrhoea, abdominal pain and fever – a disease known as 'antibiotic associated colitis'. This can be so severe that dehydration, hypotension (low blood pressure) and even perforation of the colon may occur. Check with your doctor about discontinuing the antibiotic; the colitis will generally subside by itself in 10 to 12 days, without any additional medication or treatment.

Drugs can interact with food, making the drugs work faster or slower, or preventing them from working at all. The absorption of tetracycline, a widely used antibiotic, is impaired by the calcium in dairy products. Fizzy drinks, fruit and vegetable juices with high acid content (such as orange, tomato, grape or apple) cause some drugs to dissolve in the stomach instead of the intestines where they can be more readily absorbed.

Table 5 shows a few examples of commonly used drugs with side effects that may adversely affect the digestive tract.

What you can do
If drug side effects are severe, discuss risks and benefits with your doctor, and ask if medication can be changed or the dosage

TABLE 5

SOME DRUGS FOR CHRONIC CONDITIONS

Medical use	Drug type	Some trade names	Effect on the digestive tract
Prescription Drugs:			
Antibiotic	Tetracyclines	Aureomycin Terramycin Tetracyn	Disturbance of normal gut bacteria leading to superinfection with thrush (*Candida*). Possible liver and kidney damage. Nausea, vomiting and diarrhoea. Loss of taste (possibly temporary).
Antidepressant (tricyclic)	Imipramine, Amitriptyline	Tofranil, Elavil	Dry mouth, constipation. Paralysis of large intestine. Nausea, vomiting, liver damage.

Medical use	Drug type	Some trade names	Effect on the digestive tract
Anti-inflammatory (for arthritis)	Nonsteroid	Indocin, Advil, Naprosyn	Stomach irritation. Impairment of kidneys. Possible stomach ulcers and bleeding.
	Gold salts	Ridaura, Myochrisine	Possible mouth ulcers.
	Azathioprine	Imuran	Possible nausea.
	Methotrexate	Rheumatrex	Possible liver damage.
	Dextropro-poxyphene	Darvon, Distalgesic	Nausea, vomiting, abdominal pain, constipation.
	Ibuprofen	Brufen, Motrin	Gastrointestinal haemorrhage. Nausea, vomiting, indigestion, diarrhoea.
	Indomethacin		Gastric ulceration. Stomach ulcers, nausea, vomiting, indigestion, diarrhoea.
Chronic bronchitis	Sulphon-amides	Septrin, Bactrim	Long term use may cause liver damage, mouth ulcers. Crystals of the drug may be formed in the kidney.
Heart conditions	Betablockers	Inderal, Trasicor	Nausea, vomitting, diarrhoea.
	Cardiac glycosides	Lanoxin, Digitaline	Nausea, salivation, vomiting, diarrhoea, abdominal pain.
Hypertension	Methyldopa	Aldomet	Liver damage, dry mouth, nausea, diarrhoea, constipation. Pancreatic disease, salivary gland inflammation, black tongue.
	Thiazide diuretics	Navidrex, Moduretic	Nausea.
Tranquillizers	Benzo-diazepines	Valium, Librium, Mogadon	Mouth dryness.
	Pheno-thiazines	Largactil, Thorazine, Stelazine	Mouth dryness, liver damage.
Urinary tract infections	Sulphon-amides	Septrin, Bactrim	Long term use may cause liver damage, mouth ulcers. Crystals of the drug may be formed in the kidney.

Medical use	Drug type	Some trade names	Effect on the digestive tract
Non-prescription Drugs:			
Pain relief	Aspirin		Stomach irritation and bleeding.
Coughs and colds	With sympathomi- metic drugs		Nausea, vomiting, thirst.
	With anti- histamines		Nausea, vomiting diarrhoea, constipation, colic, stomach ache, dry mouth.

modified. Read labels of non-prescription medicines for information about possible side effects and drug interactions. If in doubt, ask the chemist.

When you have a new prescription, ask your doctor:

- What is the name of the medicine, what is in the prescription, and what is it supposed to do?
- What side effects might occur, and are digestive upsets to be expected?
- Should you take the medicine before, with or after meals? Some drugs should not be taken on an empty stomach.
- Are there any foods or beverages you should avoid? Some drugs should not be taken with milk.
- Should you avoid alcohol or smoking while taking the drug?
- Are there other medicines you should not take while you are taking this one?

All medicines, whether prescription or non-prescription, should be locked up, out of the reach of children.

Travel

Travel can affect digestion, elimination, regularity of meals and regularity of bowel movements. Sitting for long periods of time can aggravate haemorrhoids. Digestive upsets can occur in four main ways: the stress induced by travel, motion sickness, jet lag and travellers' diarrhoea.

Travel stress

A holiday should be a time for relaxation and an escape from workday worries, but vacations are fraught with situations that bring on stress to churn up your stomach: getting stuck in traffic on the way to the airport, queueing to check in, worrying when the plane will leave, being afraid of flying, white-knuckled at take off and landing; and arriving at an hotel only to be told you have no reservation. Crowds, noise, strange languages, unfamiliar currencies, homesickness, different foods, drinks and lifestyles. The mind has a tendency to race the entire body, causing gas, diarrhoea, constipation and insomnia.

What you can do

- Allow extra time at every turn. Don't try to accomplish too much. Arrange the trip in such a way as to avoid a tight schedule and 'getting your money's worth'.
- Avoid taking too much luggage. If you don't over-pack, you won't have to worry about your suitcase going astray.
- Pack the day before, or even the weekend before, to prevent pre-travel jitters.
- Work half a day, on the day before a trip, to get you going at a slower pace, starting off in a calm relaxed way.
- Tuck a pack of cards or a crossword puzzle in your flight bag, in case flights get delayed.
- Your doctor can prescribe medication if you are always fearful, but it is better to train the nervous system to remain calm.
- Check back to the section on stress for further ways to relax.

Motion sickness

Nelson admitted to being seasick; Lawrence of Arabia was camel-sick; astronauts have nausea on space missions. Many people suffer motion sickness whether in cars, aboard aircraft or ships. Once you start feeling upset, the smell of food cooking, tobacco smoke, a heavy perfume, or the sight of someone else being sick can easily increase your own nausea. Heat and tight clothing can make you worse. You look pale, feel clammy, a bit dizzy, or have a headache and feel queasy. Then comes real nausea, deep breathing, cold sweats, an increased amount of saliva, then vomiting. But losing the contents of your stomach doesn't always ease the rotten feeling; you just want to be left alone to recover in peace.

Motion sickness is triggered when certain kinds of head movements signal your stomach to start feeling queasy. The trouble is caused by an over-stimulation of the balance organs in the middle ear which send messages to the brain whenever your balance is disturbed. If these messages come too fast, the brain gets overwhelmed and sickness results.

What you can do
1) Seating: On aircraft, choose a seat in line with the wings, and recline your seat as far back as possible. On trains, never sit facing backwards. On cruise ships, select a cabin amidships. Children susceptible to car sickness are usually more comfortable seated in front rather than the back.
2) Don't drink alcohol or carbonated soft drinks. Two alcoholic drinks in flight can be as potent as three on the ground. The carbonation in soft drinks can bring on a stomach ache because the decreased atmospheric pressure at 35,000 feet makes gases in the stomach and intestines 20 per cent greater in volume. Don't chew gum, which can make you swallow a lot of air.
3) Avoid eating fried, fatty or spicy foods, and foods such as beans, cabbage and onions that form gases. Eat lightly and cautiously, especially when the pilot warns of turbulence ahead.
4) On aircraft, avoid looking at the horizon, and avoid reading. Keep your eyes closed.
5) Loosen your clothing.
6) Breathe deeply. On the plane, point the overhead air blower directly at your face; on the ship, be on deck in the fresh air; in a car or train, open the window.

What the doctor can do
Your physician can prescribe motion sickness drugs. These usually belong to the group of antihistamines: cyclizine (Marezine), meclizine (Bonine) or dimenhydrinate (Dramamine), and can make you drowsy. Doctors can prescribe scopolomine combined with dexadrine, but these have severe side effects. Antihistamines, tranquillizers, sleeping and motion sickness preparations may have a 'synergistic' effect if you take them while alcohol is in your body. That is, the impact of alcohol

plus the drug is greater than the effect of each on its own.

Jet lag

When you travel to different time zones, your 'biological clock' will still follow patterns established back home. This clock or *circadian rhythm* governs your daily cycle of sleeping, waking, cell division, hormone secretion, saliva, urine excretion by volume, liver function, heart activity, fluctuations in body temperature and reactions to drugs. As many as a hundred functions show daily cycles, with each system having its own tide-like ebb and flow, peaking sometime during the day and slowing at night. The rhythm is driven by an internal chemical mechanism in part of the brain in a 25-hour cycle, with daylight synchronizing the rhythm to a 24-hour day. Apart from disturbances in sleep patterns, jet lag can affect appetite, digestion, elimination and metabolism, and cause hunger at odd hours. Disruptions of body rhythms might aggravage some medical conditions or interfere with the effectiveness of particular medications, such as the amount of insulin taken by diabetics.

Jet lag symptoms seem to be influenced by the direction in which you are going – whether east or west. Travelling east across several time zones appears to have a greater effect than going westward. Two or three days are needed for body-clock resynchronization.

What you can do

If you are on a short trip of one or two days, consider trying to maintain the schedule of your home time zone.

For longer absences, try to pre-adapt your meal times and sleep patterns a few days before the flight, to conform to the time zone at your destination point. Before a westbound flight, go to bed a few hours later than normal; for an eastbound flight go to bed several hours earlier. Some people swear by special diets, but in any case avoid overeating and drinking alcohol before flights. If possible, plan to break up very long flights with one-day 'sleepovers' en route to your final destination. Airlines serve meals convenient to flight schedules and flight attendants – you should eat according to your *personal* time clock. Eat lightly and avoid alcohol during travel and for a day or two after arrival. On the plane, drink plenty of water and fruit juices (orange or grapefruit – not tomato or vegetable juice, which may be salted, adding sodium to your system). Cut down on tea and coffee; they are mild diuretics that can induce the kidneys to release urine and increase dehydration. Alcohol is unwise, since alcohol combined with the aircraft's heat and low humidity also tends to dehydrate passengers. Dehydration dries out body fluids that aid digestion and makes it more difficult for body rhythms to adjust.

After being cooped up on a plane for much of the day, a good long walk at your destination will help to reset your biological clock and avert constipation.

What the doctor can do
He or she can prescribe medications to regulate sleep upon arrival, such as short-acting benzodiazepine. A short-acting medication is one that is quickly eliminated from the body, and has little effect during the next day to cause daytime grogginess. Don't take such medications on a plane, or take them with alcohol, or with other drugs such as antihistamines which may induce drowsiness.

Check with your doctor if you are on a strict regimen of medication and plan to travel across several time zones, making your day longer or shorter. If you are diabetic, work out your personal schedule in consultation with your doctor, and be sure to request a diabetic meal when making your reservation.

Travellers' diarrhoea

Nothing can ruin a holiday more quickly than a bout of diarrhoea. It's easy to joke about Gyppy Tummy, Delhi Belly, Montezuma's Revenge, the Aztec Two-Step, or the Trotskies . . . but it's really no laughing matter. Diarrhoea afflicts one-third of the 16 million travellers from industrialized nations who visit developing countries each year. The trouble seems to be more common among people travelling from a temperate climate to one that's more tropical. The chance of developing diarrhoea depends on the destination.

High-risk areas: Latin America, Africa, the Middle East and Southeast Asia.
Intermediate-risk areas: most of Southern Europe, Caribbean islands, the Soviet Union, and China.

Low-risk areas: Northern Europe, Australia, New Zealand, Canada and the USA.

The symptoms of diarrhoea include frequent loose stools, abdominal cramps, nausea, bloating and malaise which usually start abruptly, most often during the first week after you arrive. An attack of travellers' diarrhoea usually lasts three to four days, although 10 per cent of cases last longer than a week. A few cases persist for a month or more. Travellers' diarrhoea seems to be slightly more common in young people than in older adults, probably because youngsters are more adventurous and less careful about what they eat, and with less money to spend they can't be selective of where they eat, and may overindulge, indiscriminately drinking the local water and wine.

The most commonly identified cause of diarrhoea is *Escherichia coli*, a common species of intestinal bacteria, although other viruses, bacteria and protozoa may also be the cause.

Infection is spread through sewage-contaminated food or water. Both cooked and uncooked foods can be risky if carelessly handled. Especially dangerous are raw vegetables, leafy salads, raw meat, raw seafood, unpasteurized milk and dairy products, and unpeeled fruits. Tap water is dangerous, as are ice cubes made from local water. Freezing sharply reduces the pathogen population but does not immediately destroy the organisms responsible for diarrhoea such as *Shigella* which are more hardy. Taking water for drinking and cooking from lakes, streams and rivers contaminated by body wastes, sewage, and other sources of infectious organisms increases your risk of cholera, hepatitis, rotavirus, shigellosis and typhoid fever.

Cholera is a severe form of diarrhoea, caused by *Vibrio comma*. According to the World Health Organization, it is present in 23 countries in Asia and Africa: Angola, Benin, Burkina Faso, Burundi, Cameroon, Ghana, Guinea, India, Indonesia, Iran, Ivory Coast, Liberia, Malaysia, Mali, Mauritania, Nigeria, Rwanda, Sierra Leone, Sri Lanka, Tanzania, Thailand, Vietnam, and Zaire.

If you follow the usual tourist itineraries using standard accommodations (even in countries affected by cholera), you are at little risk of infection. But *where* you eat food is important: generally, the risk is least in private homes and good restaurants, and greatest when food comes from street vendors. If you can't boil it, cook it or peel it – forget it!

What you can do

- Avoid eating fruit with the skin already peeled.
- Make sure all meats and all vegetables are well cooked. Farmers in some developing countries still use human waste as fertilizer.
- Avoid raw oysters and other raw seafood.
- Don't drink milk or milk products unless you see the milk being boiled. Many countries do not use pasteurization.
- Drink bottled water, mineral water, boiled water, or water chemically treated with iodine or chlorine. Try to minimize swallowing water when swimming. Avoid ice cubes and iced drinks.
- Bottled carbonated drinks, beer and wine are usually safe.

How can you ward off diarrhoea? Yogurt is thought to restore normal intestinal microflora, but the culture is usually of a 'non-implantable' strain which does not survive beyond the digestive process in the stomach. The culture in sweet acidophilus milk, however, can be helpful.

A new study suggests *Bismuth subsalicylate* (the active ingredient in Pepto-Bismol) may be effective, although it will probably produce temporary side effects of blackening the tongue and darkening stools.

If travellers' diarrhoea strikes: Stop eating solid foods. Start drinking plenty of safe fluids, bottled water and tinned fruit juices. A non-medicinal method can be used to restore your body's supply of glucose and potassium and balance your system's salts depleted by dehydration:

> Take two glasses. In the first, put 8 oz fruit juice, ½ teaspoon of honey and a pinch of table salt. In the second glass, put 8 oz carbonated water or thoroughly-boiled water and ¼ teaspoon bicarbonate of soda (baking soda). Thoroughly mix the contents in each glass, then sip from each glass alternately.

What the doctor can do

Some drugs, such as entero-vioform, that were used in the past are now considered dangerous. For mild diarrhoea, prescriptions can be antimotility drugs such as diphenoxylate (Lomotil) or loperamide (Imodium). For more severe diarrhoea, there are antimicrobial drugs such as trimethoprim/sulfamethoxazole, trimethoprim alone, or doxycycline which is a broad-spectrum antibiotic. In general, however, physicians do not automatically prescribe antimicrobial drugs because although they reduce the incidence of travellers' diarrhoea, they carry the risk of serious side effects, including allergic reactions, mild and severe skin rashes, photosensitivity and blood disorders. Antimicrobial treatment may induce colitis, *Candida vaginitis* and possibly *Salmonella enteritis*.

Sexual practices

Although affecting only a small section of the population, a brief mention should be made concerning disorders that stem from certain sexual practices. Among homosexual men and some heterosexual couples, the anus-rectum is used as a sexual organ. The disorder referred to as *gay bowel syndrome* is a collection of conditions: rectal inflammation, abscesses and fistulas that resemble Crohn's disease (see Chapter 10), as well as rectal pain, diarrhoea or constipation, painful defecation, the passage of mucus and possibly bleeding.

Intimate contact involving rectum, mouth and hands can transmit infections from organisms in the intestinal tract which are more usually derived from eating or drinking faecally-contaminated food or water. Breaks in the delicate lining of the rectum allow the transfer of parasites such as *Entamoeba histolytica* and *Giardia lamblia*, viruses such as Types A and B hepatitis, and bacteria such as Salmonella and Shigella.

Consequently, it helps your doctor prescribe appropriate drug treatments if he or she is aware of your sexual preferences and habits.

PART THREE

What are the main problems?

CHAPTER 5

The mouth, teeth, gums and gullet

You may not usually associate the mouth and teeth with indigestion, but they are vital to the process of digestion. When food is not properly chewed because of difficulties in the mouth, troubles can ensue further along the gastrointestinal (GI) tract.

Cold sores (fever blisters)

These generally occur on the gums and the roof of the mouth, or on the *outside* of the lips and nostrils, and are caused by the *contagious* virus *Herpes simplex*. There are two types of Herpes simplex viruses: Herpes simplex 1 primarily causes blister-like sores on the mouth, lips and face, although these blisters can be caused by Herpes simplex 2 which is the virus that usually causes genital herpes. Herpes simplex is highly contagious when sores (fever blisters) are present, and the virus is frequently transmitted by kissing. The blisters/sores are often accompanied by fever (hence the name), swollen neck glands and general aches. Fever blisters tend to merge and then collapse. Often a yellowish crust forms over the sores, which usually heal without scarring within two weeks.

Once a person is infected with oral herpes, the virus often remains dormant in the body for a lifetime, in a nerve located near the cheekbone, either inactive or causing recurrent attacks. Outbreaks can be triggered by emotional stress, fever, illness, injury and overexposure to the sun. Some women only have recurrences during certain phases of their menstrual cycles.

What you can do

Minimize stress, and minimize sun exposure by using hats or

sun-blocking creams. Cut out rich foods such as nuts, chocolate and seeds. When a blister is forming, apply a paste of salt and water to draw out some of the fluid. After it erupts, keep it clean and dry. Non-prescription ointments reduce scab formation. A soft bland diet is less irritating to the sores and surrounding sensitive areas. To prevent spreading the virus, avoid touching sores or kissing, don't share toothbrushes, and keep toothbrushes separated.

What the doctor can do
Apply ointments that numb or that soften the crusts of the sores; provide antibiotics to control secondary infections. Some doctors recommend tablets containing *Lactobacillus acidophilus* or *L. bulgaricus*, or eating live-culture yogurt.

Mouth ulcers/canker sores

These are generally larger than cold sores, but not preceded by a blister. They are painful, but *not* contagious. They usually occur on the tongue and *inside* linings of the cheeks and lips, or at the base of the gums, showing up as round or oval yellowish-white spots with red rims. These ulcers may be hereditary, which partially explains why they tend to be shared in some families. Most of the time, they appear unrelated to diet, but 20 per cent of sufferers with frequent bouts have nutritional deficiencies, especially a lack of vitamin B_{12}, folic acid and iron. Ulcers can occur in conjunction with the inability to digest certain cereals, and might be an allergic reaction to some foods. Mouth ulcers may be caused by a faulty immune system that uses the body's defences against disease to attack and destroy the normal cells of the mouth or tongue. Women are more likely than men to have recurrent ulcers, and often only during certain phases of their menstrual cycles, with improvement during pregnancy, which suggests that female sex hormones may play a part in causing them.

What you can do
Minimize emotional stress. Avoid injuries to the mouth, such as scratching with abrasive foods or a stray toothbrush bristle that can trigger (though probably not cause) the outbreaks.

When an outbreak occurs, avoid rough foods such as potato crisps and acid and spicy foods. A weak solution of sodium bicarbonate may lessen the pain. Brush teeth carefully to avoid stabbing the ulcers with a toothbrush bristle.

What the doctor can do
Numbing preparations such as xylocaine may be prescribed to apply to the ulcers. Anti-inflammatory steroid mouthwashes or gels can be helpful if you have several ulcers. Mouthwashes containing the antibiotic tetracycline may help speed healing. For severe recurrent ulcers, you may need steroid or other immuno-suppressant drugs taken orally, under the close supervision of your physician or dentist.

Mouth dryness

This may be a side effect when taking diet pills, appetite suppressants, amphetamines and related drugs. Lack of saliva allows acids from food to increase tooth decay, food may be hard to moisten and chew, swallowing may be difficult and subsequently lead to poor digestion.

What you can do
Drink liquids frequently, and chew on pieces of chopped or crushed ice. Avoid alcohol-containing mouthwashes, since they have a drying effect. Check your prescription with your doctor, to ensure that you have the correct dosage. He may be able to change your medicine.

Change in sensitivity to taste

As you age, sensitivity to flavours and smells usually decreases, food tastes more bland, and meals are perhaps less enjoyable. If nothing tastes good, you may be using more salt or sugar on foods to combat the flat taste. You may have lost taste sensitivity because you smoke, or because of the side effects of some drugs. Temporary loss of taste can occur when the tongue is burned, or if you drink heavily, have a viral infection or an extremely bad cold.

What you can do
If taste is lost because of smoking or strong alcoholic drinks, this is one good reason for quitting. Instead of reaching for the salt

cellar, try chewing food more thoroughly; chewing breaks down food, allowing more molecules to interact with taste receptors in the mouth. Or take bites of different foods alternately; a flavour is stronger with the first bite than with subsequent ones. Perk up flavours without using salt by squeezing lemon juice or sprinkling fresh herbs over foods.

Gum disease and poor teeth

Gum disease (*gingivitis*) takes more teeth from our jaws every year than any other major dental disease, including tooth decay. Foul breath (*halitosis*) is almost always caused by diseased or infected gums, not decayed teeth. Mouthwash only temporarily trades one smell for another.

Most gingivitis starts with plaque – a colourless film made up of living and dead bacteria that constantly forms from sugars and starches in foods and collects mainly on the tooth surfaces most exposed to saliva. Dental hygienists have observed a greater build-up of dental plaque in patients that are known to be in stressful situations. Plaque turns into a deposit of tartar containing irritating toxins which cause tender, swollen, bleeding gums and which eventually push back the gumline. Some factors that contribute to gum disease, although they are not direct causes, are smoking or chewing tobacco, poor nutrition, pregnancy, diabetes or certain blood diseases, badly-aligned teeth, nail-biting, clenching or grinding the teeth, ill-fitting dentures or partial dentures, and some medications including oral contraceptives and some anti-epilepsy, steroid and cancer drugs.

Inadequate chewing can result when cavities in the teeth are left unfilled and cause so much pain that eating is avoided in certain parts of the mouth. Partially-chewed chunks of food may lodge in the throat, or hamper the digestive process in the stomach and cause elimination problems. If chewing is so painful that diet is switched to mushy foods that need little chewing, you will lack the necessary 'roughage' and end up with constipation. Biting and chewing can be affected by malocclusion, which means that there is poor alignment of the teeth so that you don't use them efficiently.

Babies are a special concern. Many parents put their babies to sleep with a bottle containing sweetened juice, milk, formula or sugar-water, causing rampant decay. This condition is often referred to as nursing-bottle-mouth, or bottle-mouth syndrome, usually seen in children aged one to four. The best idea is to give no bottle at bedtime. If you must give one, just use plain water.

What you can do
Brushing and flossing are vital for keeping gums and teeth healthy, massaging gums and removing germs and food debris. Brushing after every meal is best; brushing before bedtime is a must. A variety of foods in moderation will help ensure that you get the right balance of nutrients you need for healthy teeth. Cut back on sugar, which is a major contributor to dental cavities. Critical factors are the *amount* of sugar you eat, how *sticky* the sugar is, and *when* you eat it.

Eating sweets only at mealtime will result in less damage than sweets eaten between meals, because other foods at meals stimulate salivary flow which helps wash away food debris. Any food that stays longer in contact with teeth is more likely to cause cavities: avoid sticky toffee, jelly beans and fudge, dried fruits such as raisins and dates, and sweetened soft drinks.

What the dentist can do
She can remove plaque and tartar, perform curettage on diseased gum tissue, prescribe fluoride supplements, apply a surface sealant to reduce pit and fissure cavities, replace worn or defective fillings, remove infected pulp in teeth, correct chewing and biting problems by reshaping teeth or orthodontic treatment; apply braces, splints or other fixtures to stabilize loose teeth, provide plastic guards to control teeth-grinding when you're asleep and replace teeth with permanent surgical implants or partial dentures.

Mouth cancers

The vast majority of oral cancers occur on the floor of the mouth behind the front teeth, on the underside and sides of the tongue, and on the soft palate at the top of the mouth. Most cases of bleeding in the mouth are not cancerous, but if you have any velvety red spots, white patches or sores in the mouth that bleed or do not go away within a fortnight, be sure to have them checked by a dentist. Red or white patches on the tongue may be caused by tobacco smoking, chewing tobacco, alcohol, sharp-edged or diseased teeth or sharp-edged dentures. Another warning sign is a lump in the cheek that can be felt with the tongue. Heavy smokers who are heavy drinkers, and those with a family history of this type of cancer are at highest risk.

What you can do
Give up smoking and heavy drinking. Brush teeth and see your dentist regularly. Eat sensibly.

What the dentist or doctor can do
Mouth cancer, like any other cancer, needs to be biopsied for a definite diagnosis, by removing a small piece or the entire suspected area. Your dentist can investigate the cause and correct it, and remove patches with an electric needle, surgery, and radiation.

Swallowing problems

There can be several reasons why you may find it difficult to swallow. You may have 'a lump in your throat', for which the medical term is *globus hystericus*. This is one of the commonest symptoms of anxiety or grief, and the problem is usually overcome by just realizing it is associated with these feelings. But difficulties may also stem from muscle and nervous system disorders or problems in the oesophagus. When food 'gets stuck' on the way down, the complaint is known as *dysphagia*. Dysphagia can be the result of inflammation of the oesophagus (*oesophagitis*) when acid and gastric juices from the stomach have backed up. Oesophagitis can also result from swallowing foods and drinks that are scalding hot. Children may damage their gullets when trying to drink commercial oven cleaners, drain openers and other caustic substances. Adults attempting suicide with these same caustic substances sometimes end up surviving but unable to swallow. Swallowing may be difficult because contractile rings of tissue have formed on the inside surface of the oesophagus and narrowed the inside diameter.

What you can do

Just knowing that your difficulty in swallowing is due to anxiety or grief is sometimes sufficient for the problem to disappear. If the difficulty persists, or may have a physical cause, see your doctor.

What the doctor can do

Your physician may give you a barium meal then X-ray the oesophagus; or use a flexible fibre-optic instrument for a direct examination. A thorough examination is necessary because one cause of dysphagia is cancer of the oesophagus. The doctor may snip off tissue for biopsy if he finds contractile rings on the inside surfaces. Removing tissue may be sufficient to bring relief in swallowing.

Cancer of the oesophagus

The main symptom of oesophageal cancer is also difficulty in swallowing, dysphagia. Other warning signs of this cancer include sensations of pressure, burning or pain in the upper middle part of the chest, hoarseness, coughing, choking or fever. Because of the difficulty in swallowing, another symptom can be weight loss. Tumours start in the lining of the membrane. Most tumours of the oesophagus are malignant. More men than women have oesophageal cancer, and it occurs most often between the ages of fifty and seventy.

What the doctor can do

The first test is usually a barium-swallow followed by an X-ray. If a tumour is present, the lining of the oesophagus will appear narrowed or abormal. The physician may inspect the area with an oesophagoscope, which is a long, thin tube with a light and lens at the end of it, and remove tissue for biopsy. Cancer of the gullet is usually treated by radiation, an operation, or a combination of both.

Choking

If a piece of food misses the oesophagus and becomes stuck in the windpipe, it can stop breathing and cause unconsciousness, permanent brain damage, and/or death within four to six minutes.

Choking on food or foreign objects is the greatest cause of accidental death in the home among children under one year. Toddlers who don't chew food well can choke when they try to swallow things whole. They need supervision when eating carrot sticks, celery sticks, grapes, biscuits and nuts. For safety, cut or crumble those foods into small pieces. Cocktail sticks and toothpicks can be hazardous around children. Watch out for toothpicks holding together a club sandwich or stuffed cabbage. If swallowed accidentally, a toothpick can cause severe inflammation, puncture the bowel, or even result in death.

What you can do

First ask the person: are you choking? If the victim cannot speak, give the Heimlich Manoeuvre:

1. Stand behind the victim and wrap your arms around the person's waist.
2. Make a fist with one hand and place your fist thumb-side against the victim's stomach in the mid-line just *above* the navel and well below the rib cage.
3. Grasp your fist with your other hand.
4. Press into the stomach with a quick upward thrust. Repeat thrust, if necessary. If the manoeuvre is performed correctly, the obstruction should fly out of the mouth.

If the victim is unconscious, sweep the mouth with a finger to clear away any object or food pieces, being careful not to push the object deeper into the throat. Then attempt rescue breathing by giving abdominal thrusts until emergency help arrives:

1. Kneel and straddle the victim's hips.
2. Put the heel of one hand on the victim's abdomen, slightly above the navel and below the rib cage.
3. Put your other hand on top of the first hand and press inward and upward with six to ten quick thrusts.

If a child under eight years of age is choking, avoid finger sweeps since the object may be pushed back into the airway. Only remove objects if you can see them.

CHAPTER 6

Heartburn, hiatal hernia and vomiting

Heartburn

Eat, drink and be wary, for tonight you may have heartburn. Heartburn has nothing to do with your heart, although it can certainly feel like a fire burning in your chest. Medical experts estimate that 70 per cent of patients who come to hospital emergency rooms because they think they are having a heart attack are having a bout of heartburn.

(On the other hand, people who are really having heart attacks may delay seeking help because they believe the pain to be indigestion. If indigestion seems unusually severe and is accompanied by breathlessness, sudden nausea or vomiting, fainting, palpitations, heavy sweating or a cold clammy feeling, your 'indigestion' may be a heart attack requiring emergency treatment. You need medical help immediately.)

Doctors once blamed hiatal hernia for causing heartburn (see next section), but not all people with hiatal hernia have heartburn, and some with severe heartburn have no hiatal hernia.

Heartburn is usually your body's protest against high living. If you eat a wholesome low-fat diet as a general rule, the sudden onslaught of fats and other irritants can upset even a cast-iron stomach. Overindulgence and tensions at parties and holidays can make the problem even worse. Combine overwork with rich food and drinks, and perhaps too much coffee to help keep you going, and you've set the stage for acid indigestion. Acid indigestion can start about an hour or so after eating. It begins in the centre of your chest near the base of the breastbone, with a burning sensation that results from the back-flow of stomach acid into the oesophagus, irritating the lining of the oesophagus. Your mouth may even taste some of the hot, sour reflux. Other symptoms can be belching, a bloated feeling, or even a sore throat caused by the acid reflux. The back-flow of acid is usually the result of a drop in pressure in the lower oesophagus or a malfunction of the lower oesophageal sphincter. If the muscle loses tone, or relaxes at the wrong time, stomach acid and digestive enzymes flow back into the gullet, giving you the burning sensation.

Big meals can weaken the oesophageal sphincter; smoking and coffee are thought to relax oesophageal pressure. Susceptibility increases with age, overweight, smoking, pregnancy, stress, or with vigorous exercise. Obesity tends to increase pressures with the abdomen. If you eat while tense, angry or suffering undue stress, you can be a victim; you may feel heartburn after rushed meals during the week but have no problems when you are relaxed at the weekend. Another cause of heartburn can be restrictive clothing such as a tight belt or bra that interferes with normal distension after a meal.

Heartburn appears to be rare during the early months of pregnancy, but seems to affect about 50 per cent of all expectant mothers in the last few months of gestation. Pressure of the foetus is responsible for the reflux, and the hormone progesterone may reduce pressure of the sphincter muscle; but heartburn usually disappears after childbirth.

Bending over forward, lifting something heavy, or exercising vigorously just after a meal, can bring on heartburn. Activities such as rowing, sit-ups, weight-lifting and, to some degree, running, increase abdominal pressure, which weakens the sphincter muscle and allows the back-flow of stomach acid.

When rich, acid or spicy foods are eaten, or eaten too quickly, they trigger heartburn by irritating and stimulating acid secretion. For example:

- deep-fried, greasy, fatty anything;
- milk, cheeses and cream dips;
- tea, chocolate and coffee (including decaffeinated and acid-neutralized);
- citrus fruits, juices and tomato products;
- garlic, onions, cabbage and green peppers;

- spices and flavourings such as hot peppers, chilli powder, cumin, nutmeg, ginger, cinnamon, allspice, spearmint and peppermint. The major components of the volatile oil in peppermint trigger belching. Although peppermint oil can stimulate bile flow and can promote digestion, at the same time it affects the sphincter muscle adversely.

What you can do

If you know which foods give trouble, obviously you need to avoid them. Steer clear of after-dinner chocolate mints, peppermint sweets, mint liqueurs and peppermint teas. Avoid carbonated soft drinks, beers and sparkling wines, because the bubbles accumulate in the oesophagus and stomach, causing more distension, reflux and belching. Foods that have air incorporated into them such as soufflés, meringues, whipped cream and popcorn may also cause problems.

Eat slowly and moderately. If you feel tense, eat little or nothing until you calm down. Don't go to a party feeling ravenous, because you'll be more likely to eat everything in sight and too much of it.

Loosen clothing after eating a heavy meal.

Stop smoking; the nicotine in cigarettes reduces the tension of the sphincter muscle dramatically.

If you must bend over after a meal, bend from the knees and keep your back straight. Don't exercise immediately after eating.

Don't slump in a reclining chair after a big meal. Don't try to sleep while your stomach is full. Time your meals so that you eat at least three or four hours before bedtime. If possible, sleep in a semi-sitting position on several pillows or raise the head of the bed about six inches. The angle will help gravity keep unwanted stomach juices from flowing back.

If you are overweight, slim down.

Sucking a boiled sweet (hard candy), *not* mint-flavoured, can stimulate saliva flow to help neutralize acid irritation. Milk is not a good idea, as it stimulates stomach-acid secretions.

If acid indigestion threatens, non-prescription antacids can bring relief of meal-related heartburn by neutralizing stomach acid and soothing the oesophagus. Before you pick an antacid, talk with your doctor or pharmacist, especially if you are taking other medications. Antacid preparations may contain aspirin,

TABLE 6

A REVIEW OF ANTACIDS

Antacid	Common reactions
Sodium bicarbonate (bicarbonate of soda, baking soda)	Produces gassiness. May cause body systems to become too alkaline. May cause 'rebound' of stomach acid production. Sodium may cause water retention and hypertention, leading to kidney and heart problems.
Calcium carbonate	Constipation. Can assist calcium absorption and bone metabolism. Overuse can lead to high calcium levels in blood which may cause increased acid production.
Magnesium oxide or magnesium hydroxide (Milk of Magnesia)	Diarrhoea. Undesirable retention of magnesium which can be serious for people with kidney disease.
Aluminium hydroxide	Constipation or diarrhoea. Can block calcium and fluoride absorption, which alters bone metabolism.

Note: Non-prescription antacids may contain any of the above or a combination of them, plus aspirin, and may be in liquid or tablet form.

which should not be taken needlessly, particularly if you have other gastrointestinal problems.

Some people take bicarbonate of soda (baking soda), and many antacids are primarily composed of sodium bicarbonate. Bicarbonate neutralizes acid in the stomach temporarily, and, by creating carbon dioxide gas, provides enough gas to permit belching. But if you must restrict your intake of salt or sodium because of problems such as high blood pressure, a heart condition or fluid-retention, choose a low-sodium antacid. See *The Salt-Watcher's Guide* (Thorsons, 1986).

Liquid antacids, although not always the most convenient, can help to wash the acid back to where it belongs and are usually more effective than the chewable variety, which should be chewed very thoroughly. About a tablespoon of a liquid antacid is as effective as three tablets of the same antacid.

Whether liquid or tablet, most non-prescription antacids have a combination of ingredients, including sodium bicarbonate, calcium carbonate, aluminium hydroxide and magnesium hydroxide. See the antacid review in Table 6.

Antacids are best taken between meals, at bedtime and at least an hour before or after taking other medications. Some antacids can cause occasional side effects, such as diarrhoea, constipation, altered calcium metabolism and magnesium retention. Chronic use of antacids containing aluminium compounds may seriously deplete your body and bone structure of calcium; aluminium interferes wtih the absorption of fluoride and can contribute to skeletal demineralization. See *Brittle Bones and the Calcium Crisis* (Thorsons, 1987). Antacids combined with a foaming agent such as alginic acid may be helpful. These compounds are believed to form a foam barrier on the top of the gastric pool.

To relieve pregnancy-related heartburn, eating small meals more frequently is often helpful. Doctors sometimes prescribe antacids that promote renewal of acid-damaged tissue, but not medicines that work by entering the system to suppress acid production.

If it becomes necessary to use non-prescription antacids for longer than three weeks, see your doctor.

What the doctor can do

If the burning symptoms persist or the pain is very severe, you have difficulty swallowing, food seems to stick in your chest, or if the chest pain doesn't fit heartburn's description, you should consult your physician. Heartburn more than three or four times a week can cause inflammation, scarring and constriction of the oesophagus, and may even eventually make conditions conducive to cancer, or you could have symptoms of a peptic ulcer.

For serious heartburn, some doctors prescribe drugs such as ranitidine and cimetidine which work by suppressing the gastric acid secretion instead of neutralizing it. Or the doctor can increase pressure of the oesophageal sphincter with drugs such as bethanechol or metoclopramide, or perform surgery to strengthen the sphincter.

Hiatal Hernia

In former times, many people believed that heartburn was a result of having a hiatal hernia. While heartburn is sometimes associated with hiatal hernia, it is not caused by it. Hiatal hernia occurs when a portion of the stomach protrudes through a hole in the diaphragm where the oesophagus and the stomach join. The most frequent causes are coughing, vomiting, straining at a bowel movement, sudden exertion, pregnancy or being overweight.

What you can do
Lose weight, if that is the cause of the problem. Improve your diet with more fibre to avoid straining at bowel movements; see the section on dietary fibre on page 34.

What the doctor can do
Most hiatal hernias do not need treatment, but if the oesophagus becomes inflamed, or the hernia is in danger of becoming constricted to cut off blood supply, your doctor can perform surgery to reduce the size of the hernia.

Vomiting

Vomiting – the violent emptying of the stomach – may have a physical or a psychological cause. Vomiting (*emesis*) can be triggered by contaminated food, by poisons or drugs such as aspirin, syrup of ipecacuanha, digitalis and some antibiotics. Sometimes an allergy to foods may cause sudden vomiting. Or it may be due to infections, gastritis, alcohol hangover, kidney diseases, gastrointestinal cancer (and the chemotherapy and radiation used in cancer treatments), peptic ulcers, bowel obstructions, appendicitis, inflammations of the gallbladder and pancreas, liver diseases, migraine headaches and pregnancy.

Vomiting often occurs with other symptoms, which can help a doctor in diagnosis. For instance, when a viral disorder, infection or hangover is the cause, diarrhoea often occurs as well; heart attacks usually occur with vomiting and chest pain; brain tumour symptoms can be an intense headache accompanied by vomiting; a blow on the head may induce vomiting and may indicate swelling of the brain, or bleeding within the skull; and when children cough excessively, they may also vomit.

Vomiting can be induced by inserting a finger deep into the throat to trigger the emptying of the stomach contents – the practice of people who are desperately trying to remain slim or bulimics in their bouts of gorging and purging.

When you vomit, the vomiting centre in the brain (the *medulla oblongata*, which also regulates breathing and heartbeat), is stimulated by certain events that lead to the expulsion of the stomach contents through the mouth. A signal is transmitted through nerve fibres to the vagus and other nerves in the pharynx, larynx, stomach, chest wall and diaphragm. This message stimulates the heavy release of saliva, causes blood to drain from the face, lowers blood pressure and heart rate, and slows gastric motility or stops it altogether. At the same time, the pyloric sphincter in the stomach closes and the lower oesophageal sphincter and oesophagus muscles relax. A strong contraction of the abdominal muscles pumps the gastric content up through the oesophagus and forcefully ejects it from the mouth as *vomitus*.

The vomiting centre in the brain is sensitive to emotional stimuli, though this susceptibility varies considerably among individuals: some people have 'strong stomachs' and seldom vomit; others find they are more sensitive, and can have a lifelong problem of gastric instability.

The vomiting centre may respond to stress, fear or depression, sudden shock or fright, when for instance people are involved in horrible accidents or fires, are raped or violently attacked, are experiencing difficulties in marriage or the death of a loved one. Emotional upsets can literally make people sick.

Children sometimes use deliberate vomiting as an expression of defiance against parents, as a weapon to avoid going to school, or as a fearful response to the first day of school. Repeated vomiting without physical cause is often seen among children exposed to child abuse. The problem can become chronic when a child realizes that sickness can provoke anger or concern in others or is a means of getting increased attention.

Vomiting is frequently preceded by nausea, when the stomach seems to 'turn over', you have a feeling of being repelled by food, the smell of food or tobacco, and an urgent need to vomit – although actual vomiting may not occur. Nausea can be brought on by unpleasant smells or unpleasant sights such as seeing a bad cut, injury or the sight of blood. Nausea is almost always relieved by vomiting, but sometimes nothing is expelled from the stomach and the result is only retching – strong muscular contractions of the abdomen and chest.

Chronic psychogenic vomiting may happen after any meal and tends to run in cycles of a few weeks. Sufferers of emotional vomiting may be helped by psychological counselling when the victim realizes the possible link between physical symptoms and emotional problems.

It is important to note the content of vomitus: if there is a distinctly sour taste and stinging sensation in the throat, the contents are gastric juice or bile, and this is a sign of hyperacidity or a duodenal ulcer. The presence of mucus in vomitus is common in those who have chronic gastritis, or morning sickness in pregnancy. If vomiting is violent or prolonged, or there is unproductive retching, the vomitus may contain thin streaks of blood from minute tears in the oesophagus and stomach lining. However, more than just 'streaks' of blood can be a serious warning of internal haemorrhage. Vomiting of blood (haematemesis) is serious, and requires an immediate professional medical examination. Pus in vomitus may signal a gastric abscess and medical help should be sought promptly.

What you can do
Lie down with a cool damp cloth on the forehead and avoid solid food. Relax, and try deep breathing until the feeling of nausea passes. Replace fluids lost with vomiting by sipping water, or simple broth, jelly or apple purée adding milk and milk products if they can be tolerated.

If nausea and vomiting persist for more than a day, or are

accompanied by unusual pains, or are without apparent cause, consult your doctor.

If vomiting is related to drinking too much alcohol, the symptom should subside, and what you need is time. If nausea and vomiting is associated with pregnancy, check the Pregnancy section in Chapter 4 (page 56). If vomiting is caused by motion sickness, check the Travel section in Chapter 4 (page 63).

Some cases of nausea and vomiting are related to simple constipation, if there has been no bowel movement for some time. However, persistent vomiting, abdominal distension and constipation may indicate an intestinal blockage for which professional medical attention is necessary.

What the doctor can do

Nausea and vomiting may be a side effect of prescription or non-prescription medicine you are taking for other diseases or conditions. Consult your doctor and perhaps the dosage or type of drug can be changed.

If your doctor considers that vomiting may be of psychogenic origin, treatment by psychotherapy may be suggested.

Cancer patients on chemotherapy may experience nausea and vomiting that is of short duration, or that lasts about a day, or they may have a feeling of nausea which always seems to be present. To control chemotherapy-related vomiting, the doctor can prescribe antiemetic drugs. Some cancer patients also have success in controlling nausea and vomiting with the use of hypnosis, relaxation, biofeedback and other mind-control techniques to relieve anxiety.

CHAPTER 7

Problems with the stomach

Borborygmus

Rumbles, gurgles and bubbling sounds have occurred to most of us at one time or another – probably at quiet moments at cocktail parties, to the acute embarrassment of the person whose stomach is making the sounds. Stomach rumbling is usually just a minor cause of social awkwardness, and one which can be averted or controlled, rather than a medical problem.

Gases can occur anywhere along the gastrointestinal tract. They can be due to swallowing air while talking rapidly and excitedly, drinking effervescent liquids, breathing erratically and nervously, or smoking cigarettes; or they can be generated within the system from foods you have eaten. If these gases are not eventually belched up, or passed along the intestine to be expelled as *flatus*, the movements within become audible. See also Flatulence in Chapter 10 (page 118).

The term 'empty stomach' is commonly used, but it is a misnomer because the stomach in its natural state cannot be entirely empty: it still contains gastric juices, mucus, swallowed saliva, plus any air that may have been swallowed. A growling stomach is simply indicating that it wants to be fed. When it has no food to work on, the muscles contract at irregular intervals producing 'hunger pangs'; nerve centres in the brain send signals to the stomach nerves to agitate the liquid contents with muscular movements.

Borborygmus can also occur after eating food to which the flavour-enhancer monosodium glutamate (MSG) has been added. Glutamic acid is found in human nerve tissue and plays a role in the transmission of nerve impulses, and it is believed that a temporary dietary excess may disrupt parts of the nervous system. If you are sensitive to this compound, and have a large enough dose on an empty stomach, you can develop gurgles, a feeling of pressure behind the forehead and eyes, or chest pain – the so-called 'Chinese restaurant syndrome'.

What you can do
The simplest way to avoid borborygmus is to eat regularly, eat slowly and carefully. If a meal is not immediately possible, have a mini-snack such as a small biscuit, a cracker or a sweet. It can also be helpful to drink a glass of water. If your stomach growls because of ingesting MSG, omit this substance in recipes, avoid buying ready-processed foods that may contain it, and be sure that restaurant dishes are prepared without the additive.

Gastritis

The suffix '-itis' in medical terms indicates inflammation; thus gastritis means the inflammation of the stomach, including lesions of the stomach wall, deterioration of the mucosa, and bleeding which can be microscopic or heavy. Gastroenteritis is inflammation of the lining of both the stomach and the small intestine.

Gastritis can have a number of causes: alcohol, smoking, drug use, and certain foods that damage, inflame or wear away the gastric mucosa. The reflux of intestinal contents into the stomach has been determined a cause; and genetic factors can predispose certain people to be victims. Gastritis affecting the gastric antrum section is found among people infected with the bacteria C. *pylori*, but unfortunately there is no cure yet for this infection.

If you are taking aspirin for your heart, you probably should not take aspirin for a headache, which may increase stomach inflammation. If your doctor recommends aspirin therapy for preventing a second heart attack, or if you have unstable angina, it may not be a good idea to take additional aspirin for everyday aches and pains such as headaches, muscle aches, colds or flu symptoms. Never begin such aspirin therapy without being under a doctor's supervision; let your doctor determine the dosage. Follow instructions carefully, since taking more aspirin than your doctor recommends may put you at a greater risk of stomach irritation. Sometimes serious stomach inflammation can occur without obvious symptoms, so that you may not even be aware of a problem. Read non-prescription labels to be sure that aspirin is not part of the compound. An alternative to aspirin for minor aches and pains can be acetaminophen, but first consult your physician.

Ageing produces many cases of gastritis, and women are affected more than men, but there is no typical person who may suffer, and the disease is still regarded as somewhat of an enigma. Gastritis can attack people who are calm or, on the other hand, not affect people who abuse their digestive systems.

Doctors usually divide gastritis into two main categories: acute and chronic, with the acute form of inflammation being further divided according to the cause. Thus there is alcoholic gastritis (in the vast majority of cases), corrosive gastritis and toxic gastritis.

Alcoholic gastritis

This is the result of alcohol in drinks coming in contact with the gastric mucosa, and it is estimated that 50 per cent of constant drinkers are affected by acute gastritis. Why does gastritis attack some alcoholics and not others? It appears to be a matter of individual susceptibility, probably influenced by cirrhosis of the liver, ageing, simultaneously taking medicines such as aspirin, or accompanying diseases such as diabetes, pancreatitis and tuberculosis.

Alcohol interferes with the normal mucosal barrier that protects the stomach from digesting itself. Loss of the thin, protective coating can occur with either mild or strong alcoholic solutions. When the coating is damaged, additional alcohol, acid, and all other irritants come into contact with the sensitive stomach wall, making inflammation more likely.

Alcohol increases the muscular movements of the stomach and the production of secretions. A small amount of alcohol over a long period produces only a slight change; but steady heavy drinking or a short-lived binge can create severe inflammation and haemorrhage from the mucosa.

Salicylates, such as aspirin, compound the problem, especially when taken as a 'cure' for hangover. A combined attack on the stomach wall by alcohol and aspirin is worse than either substance alone, and alcohol increases the ability of aspirin to induce bleeding.

Symptoms of alcoholic gastritis are usually first noticed on 'the morning after', waking up to nausea and pain, heaviness or fullness in the upper abdomen. Vomiting may be flecked with blood, and any bowel movements produce stools also streaked with red. Ill effects can last four or five days. Among chronic alcoholics, it is common to have profuse haemorrhage when vomit material is heavily bloody.

What you can do

Stop drinking, and allow the mucosa to heal itself – which usually takes four or five days. Avoid aspirin. Stop eating for a while, and rest. You can help healing by keeping to a light diet as soon as you can tolerate food: clear broths and soups, mashed potatoes, rice puddings and simple gelatines. A liquid antacid or bicarbonate of soda may hasten the healing process and reduce bleeding.

What the doctor can do

When bleeding is heavy, or if bloody vomiting occurs suddenly without any prior gastric symptoms, these can be danger signals and you need an examination immediately by your physician. You will need a hospital stay to have the stomach lining washed or, possibly in severe cases, have surgery with a portion of the stomach or vagus nerve removed.

Corrosive gastritis

If you accidentally (or deliberately) swallow a caustic substance such as lye or acid, it does not usually reach the stomach but results in severe inflammation or damage to the oesophagus with difficulties in swallowing, producing obstructive scar tissue. But when the caustic material affects the stomach, the consequences are far more serious than alcohol, creating destruction not only of the mucosal barrier but also the underlying layers.

You immediately have intense suffering: a burning throat, stomach pain, difficulty in swallowing, a swollen tongue, hiccups, coughing, vomiting, gastric bleeding, fever and an increased heart rate.

The mucosal barrier can also be worn away by other milder caustics such as fiery or highly-seasoned foods eaten continually. Gastritis is not caused by foods and drinks that are too hot in *temperature*, since by the time these reach the stomach they have ceased to be hot enough to affect the stomach. But culprits among condiments can be mustard, pepper, horseradish, chilli powder, curry, paprika, cloves, garlic, vinegar, pickles, vinegary salad dressings, as well as strong tea and quinine water (tonic).

Other causes of corrosive gastritis are drugs, and particularly aspirin, especially when taken on an 'empty stomach'. Your doctor may prescribe medications for other illnesses, such as antibiotics or those for arthritis, and these can have an inflammatory effect. It is important to clearly understand instructions about prescription or non-prescription medicines and whether they should be taken before, with, or after meals or a small snack.

What you can do
Store lye and acids under lock and key. If the victim has accidentally or deliberately swallowed lye, or if the substance is unknown, this is an emergency when it is *essential* to see the doctor. In most cases, *nothing* should be given by mouth, and vomiting should *not* be induced. If you know that the caustic was an acid, then milk, Milk of Magnesia, or egg white may help neutralize it. If the corrosive gastritis is diet-related, and fiery foods are to blame, by avoiding these offenders the mucosa usually heals itself within a few days.

What the doctor can do
Treatment will depend on the severity of the injury to the stomach. If the stomach wall is in danger of perforation or is severely weakened, stomach pumping is not usually performed. The doctor may give antibiotics if an infection is suspected, or treatment may include surgery.

Toxic gastritis

Swallowing poison by accident, or by intent, can affect the gastric mucosa depending on the toxin involved. Common poisonous substances found in most households include ammonia, dry-cleaning fluids, lighter fuel and petrol, rat poison, insecticides and pesticides. Symptoms will vary according to the poison swallowed but frequently include abdominal pain, nausea, vomiting, heavy salivation, perspiration, delirium and coma. The outcome is often death eventually.

Gastritis that results from eating contaminated food can be just as serious as swallowing a poison. See the Unsafe Food section in Chapter 3 (page 43).

What you can do
Prevent accidents. Carefully store all household cleaners and other potential poisons, keeping them well away from children. Do not transfer poisons to other containers which formerly held foods or beverages. Call your doctor, police, rescue squad, paramedics or poison centre immediately you have an emergency. Do not induce vomiting if the poison is petrol, paraffin or kerosene, paint solvents or cleaning fluid. Poison survivors need a bland diet during the stomach's self-healing process.

Chronic gastritis

Frequent bouts of heavy drinking expose the gastric mucosa to the constant irritation of alcohol, leading to permanent damage. Chronic gastritis occurs three times more frequently in people who have diabetes than it does in the general population. If you have been suffering diabetes mellitus for many years, an expected result is stomach irritation and inflammation. The incidence is also high in families of diabetics, and in the relatives of those with thyroid diseases and pernicious anaemia.

Chronic gastritis has a high incidence in people over the age of sixty, and some doctors believe it may be a normal component of the ageing process. The disease is common in people who are very nervous and tense, and among the emotionally unstable, in which case it usually occurs with ulcers. Many sufferers of chronic gastritis have no symptoms at all, although some people may have dull aches, pains and cramps, or bloated feelings, along with heartburn and belching.

What you can do
The usual therapy is a bland diet and frequent mini-meals instead of two or three heavy meals per day. Liquid antacids are

often helpful. Doctors usually recommend cutting out alcohol, smoking, aspirin and caffeine.

Hyperacidity

The best known symptom of hyperacidity is probably heartburn. A normal part of digestion is the production of hydrochloric acid by parietal cells in the stomach wall, and secretion of acid is stimulated by external substances such as protein, caffeine, alcohol and nicotine. A balancing factor to curb gastric acid secretion is the hormone secretin and other hormones that control stomach acid under varying conditions. When the natural balance is disrupted, the disease has often altered the population of parietal cells in the gastric mucosa. An *increase* of parietal cells is linked with ulcers in the *duodenum*; a *decrease* of these cells is associated with *gastric* ulcers, gastritis, pernicious anaemia and stomach cancer.

Your emotional state may bring about an increase in stomach acid, although studies of the problem appear to be conflicting. Well-known sufferers of hyperacidity are hard-driving businessmen; when people are faced with problems, there can be measurable increases in stomach acid. On the other hand, deep sadness, despair and feelings of futility appear to result in a decrease of both acid production and gastric muscular contractions. Hyperacidity can be the springboard to duodenal ulcers, which are described in the next chapter.

What you can do
Cut drinking and smoking. Drink coffee or tea in moderation. Refer to the Stress section in Chapter 4 (page 52) for ways to reduce tensions and anxiety.

Stomach cancer

Unfortunately the symptoms of stomach cancer are often vague and non-specific, but the most common is indigestion, including heartburn and belching, loss of appetite, nausea, fullness or bloating. These are signs that are easy to ignore, or dismiss as simple indigestion, but if they persist – even intermittently – for about a fortnight, you need to consult your doctor. Later symptoms might include dark, bloody stools, vomiting, rapid weight loss and severe pain (but these signs may also indicate the presence of an ulcer).

Cancer of the stomach can progress in stages: early detection may find the tumour confined to the lining and connective tissue of the stomach; then it involves the stomach wall; later, the tumour penetrates the stomach wall and invades nearby tissue; finally, it spreads from the stomach wall to nearby structures, invading the liver and other organs.

Doctors speculate whether stomach ulcers lead to stomach cancer. Most physicians consider that the danger of stomach ulcers lies not so much in the possibility that an ulcer may lead to malignancy, but that it may be cancerous even while being treated as an ulcer.

What you can do
Don't hesitate to see your physician for an examination if 'indigestion' persists for a week or two, or if bloody stools appear.

What the doctor can do
A careful physical and rectal examination is made, with analysis of the acidity of stomach contents and red/white blood cell count. A barium X-ray is the most important diagnostic method, and exfoliate cytology allows an examination of cells scraped from the lining of the stomach, to determine if malignant cells are present.

Depending on the location of the tumour, the usual treatment is prompt surgical removal of the malignancy, which may involve taking away a part or all of the stomach. A person can adjust quite successfully after removal of the entire stomach, by learning to eat smaller meals, more frequently, and more slowly.

Stomach cancers are usually considered resistant to treatment by radiation since a dose that would be safe for the surrounding normal tissues is not strong enough to destroy the cancer. However, it may be possible in some cases to implant radioactive material into a malignant tumour for pain relief when cancers are inoperable.

CHAPTER 8

Peptic ulcers

Sir William Osler, the great diagnostician (1849–1919), described an ulcer as the 'wound' stripe of Western civilization'. Only seventy cases were known to exist in England during the entire nineteenth century.

What is a *peptic ulcer*? It is a small sore, lesion or deep cavity that occurs in the lining of the oesophagus at its lower end, in the lining of the stomach or the lining of the duodenum, the first part of the small intestine leading from the stomach. It looks similar to a tiny crater or a minute volcano, surrounded by an inflamed area, and in fact it is sometimes referred to as an *ulcer crater*. The usual size varies from 6mm up to 50mm (¼ inch up to 2 inches) in diameter.

Peptic ulcers are non-malignant, and are found only in those areas of the digestive tract that are bathed by digestive juices secreted by the stomach. These juices contain hydrochloric acid and the digestive enzyme pepsin – hence the name 'peptic' ulcer. Peptic ulcers that appear in the stomach are called *gastric* ulcers; those that occur in the duodenum are called *duodenal* ulcers. Duodenal ulcers tend to be smaller than stomach ulcers and heal more quickly. In the USA, duodenal ulcers are more common than the gastric ones; the reverse is true in Japan. See Figure 3.

Causes

The underlying cause of ulcers is still unknown, but researchers believe that peptic ulcer disease is a group of disorders sharing the same symptom – an inflammation and destruction of tissue

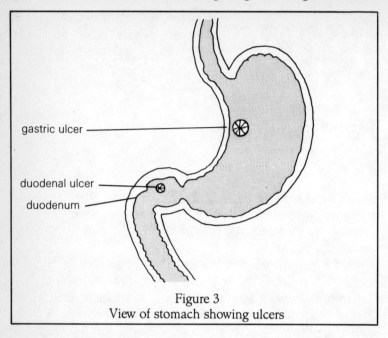

gastric ulcer

duodenal ulcer

duodenum

Figure 3
View of stomach showing ulcers

in a very localized area of the lining of the stomach or duodenum. They are sores that penetrate the lining and the muscular coat of the stomach and intestine, and maybe the wall of the bowel (perforation). An ulcer in the lower oesophagus – which is less common – can occur as a result of chronic heartburn and the regurgitation of food mixed with the stomach acid, due to a weakened sphincter or a hiatal hernia. The severity of an ulcer depends upon how deep it is and how many of the stomach's layers it penetrates.

In a healthy person, there is a balance between the amount of acid and pepsin the stomach secretes, and the ability of the lining of the stomach and duodenum to resist the erosive action of the acid and pepsin. Sometimes the balance can be upset, however, and may lead to the development of an ulcer. High acidity combined with very small amounts of pepsin makes pure gastric juice one of the most corrosive of the body's secretions. Ulcers in the duodenum are linked with an increase in the number of acid-producing parietal cells, so most people with duodenal ulcers, and some people with gastric ulcers, secrete excess amounts of pepsin and acid, which overcome the lining defences of the stomach or duodenal wall. However, some ulcer patients secrete normal amounts of gastric acid but the lining of their stomach or duodenum has a decreased resistance and is unable to tolerate these normal amounts of acid.

Symptoms

Stomach ulcers may or may not have any symptoms. Some peptic ulcers are discovered by chance during an X-ray of the upper digestive tract performed for some other reason. However, when symptoms do occur, a duodenal ulcer usually produces a gnawing or burning pain in the abdomen between the navel and the lower end of the breastbone. The pain occurs most often 1 to 1½ hours after meals and in the early hours of the morning when the stomach increases its acid secretion, and can last a few minutes to a few hours, usually relieved by eating food or taking an antacid. A gastric ulcer produces pain about 30 minutes after meals. But some people may have an ulcer with little or no pain, or they have an unrelated disorder that causes similar symptoms. Ulcer victims may have hidden or slow bleeding, with weakness as the only symptom; other people may have sudden brisk bleeding with black, tarry stools or bloody vomit, and these are emergency signals.

Ulcers can occur at any age. They are rare among children, and only slightly more common in teenagers. Duodenal ulcers usually first appear in people during their twenties or thirties, while gastric ulcers are more likely to develop among people in their forties or older. Duodenal ulcers are more common in men. Gastric ulceration affects both sexes with equal frequency (except in Australia, where a high incidence in women appears to correlate with aspirin intake).

Genetic factor

Heredity is a factor in the incidence of peptic ulcer disease which can be a family affair. Your risk for getting an ulcer is increased threefold if any of your blood relatives have ulcers; you have a greater chance of getting a duodenal ulcer if the relative has one too. Similarly, a gastric ulcer is more likely to occur if your parent or a sibling has a gastric ulcer.

Geographic factor

Researchers have found vast variations in susceptibility in different countries, and in different regions of the same country, which may be linked to genetics. Acute perforations of ulcers occur twice as often in Aberdeen, Scotland as in York, England. There is a high incidence of ulcers in southern India; a low occurrence in northern India. Among Scandinavians, there is low incidence in Swedes and Finns; a high occurrence in Danes and Norwegians. Chinese in mainland China have a low incidence of ulcers; but there is a high rate among Chinese living on the island of Java. There are differences between Chinese and Indian peoples on Java; between peoples of northern and southern Nigeria.

Where there is a high ulcer rate, the explanation may lie not only in heredity but in different eating patterns. Research using laboratory animals has shown that diets deficient in protein and vitamins A, B and C can produce stomach erosion, and this theory is borne out by studies of population groups.

Blood group factor

Researchers have also noted variations in ulcer incidence associated with the distribution of blood groups among peoples (another genetic link); those with blood type O are about 35 per cent more liable to develop duodenal ulcers than people with groups A, B and AB. Blood type O is thought to be linked with an overproduction of parietal cells. Patients with blood type O have a greater risk of haemorrhage and perforation of ulcers. Gastric ulcers are not linked as strongly with people of any particular blood type, although group A is slightly more common. It appears that a protective substance called 'AB antigen' is secreted in saliva and other gastric juices in about 80 per cent of people, regardless of blood type, and this is believed to strengthen the barrier against acid and pepsin. People with blood type O who do *not* secrete AB antigens are about twice as likely to develop ulcers as those who do.

Ulcers in women

In the countries where the incidence of ulcers has been studied, the conclusion has been that women develop the disorder far less frequently than men. Women generally have fewer parietal cells than men, and therefore a lower producion of acid. Oestrogen hormones, too, appear to offer women some protection to make them less vulnerable to ulcer development (perhaps similar to the way that oestrogens protect women from heart disease). According to studies of Scottish women with ulcers, the variations in hormonal levels during the menstrual cycle have little influence on the aggravation of existing ulcers or the formation of new ones. But during pregnancy, when oestrogen levels in blood increase a thousand times over pre-pregnancy levels, ulcers are retarded or less active. Ulcer symptoms clear up dramatically at an early stage of pregnancy – but often recur three to six months after childbirth. Around menopause, when female sex hormones diminish, bringing a diminution of all body secretions, the rate of developing new ulcers increases, or existing ulcers are aggravated.

Ulcers in children

When ulcers occur in children, they are often in families where one or more close relatives – parents, brothers and sisters – have the disorder, and a considerably higher percentage of youngsters with the disease have blood type O. Another contributory factor may be a stressful environment in the home or school creating tensions and anxiety, where parents or teachers demand perfection or strong discipline, where there is sibling rivalry, or in broken homes where emotions are high. Researchers speculate that the development of ulcers in children may be due not so much to large amounts of hydrochloric acid and pepsin but to immature or defective defensive mechanisms. Children with peptic ulcer have a high incidence of bleeding and perforation, possibly because the cause may not be recognized until these complications develop. Consequently in a family with a history of peptic ulcers, parents should consider the possibility of ulcers in their children when they complain of abdominal pain. When children are too tiny and too young to make their pain problems understood, complications are extremely serious: haemorrhage and perforation may occur following a major illness such as meningitis, a major burn, infection or congenital heart disease.

Diet

There is no convincing evidence to show that certain diets can cause ulcers (apart from the protein and vitamin deficiencies noted earlier), or that certain diets can heal ulcers and keep them healed. A diet may help relieve the pain or indigestion caused by an existing ulcer, but it will not prevent an ulcer from forming. Many foods that initially neutralize acid in the stomach, such as milk, may stimulate additional acid secretion.

Coffee and caffeine

Coffee (including decaffeinated), tea, cola soft drinks, and other foods that contain caffeine, can stimulate acid secretion in the digestive tract and may aggravate the pain of an existing ulcer. However the role of caffeine products in contributing to the development of ulcers is unknown. The level of acid secretion induced by decaffeinated coffee is the same as with regular coffee, therefore some substance other than caffeine is present in coffee to stimulate gastric action.

Alcohol

Although alcohol is often thought to be a stimulant of stomach acid secretion, numerous studies have failed to establish such a link between acid secretion and concentrated alcohol. However many alcoholics may have a poor diet and suffer degrees of malnutrition, drink a lot of coffee, smoke cigarettes and take aspirin for hangovers; these can all be contributing factors in the development of ulcers. Alcohol intensifies the effect of caffeine on gastric secretion and may increase acid production when alcohol and coffee are consumed at the same time. If you already suffer a gastric ulcer, a small amount of alcohol may be sufficient to trigger stomach bleeding.

Smoking

Cigarette smoking not only doubles your chance of getting an ulcer, but also tends to slow the healing process if you do get one. Smoking is an important factor in causing ulcer recurrence. People who stop smoking have a lower rate of recurrent ulcers regardless of what medication they may take. The chances of an ulcer healing and staying healed are better if the victim quits smoking and takes no medicine than if the patient continues to smoke and receives drug treatment.

Aspirin

In the USA, vast quantities of aspirin are taken every year; it is estimated that the British take 20 per cent more aspirin than Americans, and Australians take *twice* as much aspirin as the British. Aspirin for headaches, heart attack prevention, minor pains or arthritis (and non-steroidal anti-inflammatory drugs for arthritis) taken over long periods of time – whether taken intermittently or continuously – definitely damages the stomach lining, giving an increased risk of developing a gastric ulcer. Aspirin and similar drugs inhibit the stomach's production of substances called *prostaglandins*. Prostaglandins may act to protect the lining of the stomach from injury by the stomach's own acid secretions and other chemical agents. In most cases, these drug-related ulcers disappear once the damaging medicines are stopped.

Stress

Is peptic ulcer disease most prevalent among high-powered business executives? And as women climb the corporate and economic ladders, will their new role in Western society cancel out some of the advantage conferred on them by oestrogens and affect the rate at which they develop ulcers? The answers to these questions seem to depend on how much your body reacts to anxiety. Although stress may aggravate the pain or create indigestion associated with an ulcer, scientists have not yet been able to prove that stress is an important factor in the cause of ulcers. Doctors have noted that some patients have flare-ups during the week; less so on Sunday and Monday. Is there a link between personal stress or national crisis and ulcer development? In World War II, an increase of cases of perforated peptic ulcers was reported at Charing Cross Hospital in London during the first two months of heavy air raids in September and October 1940. In Germany the incidence of new ulcers almost doubled each year between 1938 and 1940, compared to the rate for 1937 to 1938. Wartime in Austria, Belgium, Denmark, Holland, Sweden, Switzerland, and the USA saw an increased frequency in the development of ulcers and increased numbers of cases of complications. Stress is difficult to measure, because people react differently to similar circumstances; a situation that may stress one person may have no effect on someone else. However, some ulcer patients are apparently less able to tolerate large amounts of stress or tension, and these people have said that their ulcer 'acts up' when they are confronted by emotional stress.

Physical stress, however, is definitely associated with an increase in ulcer incidence, due to greater activity of the vagus nerve; thus burns, a broken leg, surgery, and other trauma often need rigorous treatment of acidity.

Table 7 summarizes some of the differences between duodenal and gastric ulcers.

Complications

If an ulcer is left untreated, the three main serious complications are *bleeding, perforation* and *obstruction*. As an ulcer erodes the muscular portion of the gastric or duodenal wall, it can cut into blood vessels and cause bleeding into the digestive tract. If the damaged blood vessels are small, the blood may seep out slowly and, over a long period of time, you can gradually become anaemic. But if, on the other hand, a damaged blood vessel is large, bleeding is more rapid and can be very dangerous. You will feel faint, vomit blood or collapse suddenly. Some bleeding ulcers result in stools that are tarry black in colour due to the blood they contain. Without prompt medical treatment, blood transfusions and surgery, you could bleed to death.

When an ulcer erodes all the way through the stomach or duodenal wall, this perforation results in partially digested food and bacteria from the digestive tract spilling into the abdominal cavity and causing *peritonitis*, an inflammation of the abdominal cavity and wall. A perforated ulcer, which can cause sudden severe pain, usually needs a hospital stay and corrective surgery.

When an ulcer occurs in the duodenum, or in the narrow section where the stomach connects to the duodenum, this can

TABLE 7

SOME DIFFERENCES BETWEEN DUODENAL AND GASTRIC ULCERS

Duodenal ulcer	Gastric ulcer
Occurs in younger people.	Tends to occur in older persons.
Fairly intermittent pain.	Pain fairly steady.
Pain between meals or when stomach is empty.	Pain with or soon after meals.
Pain through to the back.	Pain at back is uncommon.
Nausea and vomiting uncommon.	Nausea, bloating, vomiting and belching common.
Predominantly linked with greater than normal amounts of acid.	Usually linked with normal or less than normal amounts of acid.
High incidence in persons with blood type O.	High incidence in people with blood group type A.
Tends to be in higher social classes.	Tends to be in lower social groups.
Linked with highly-anxious people in intellectually-demanding jobs.	Linked with jobs of heavy physical labour.
Eating a snack relieves symptoms.	Foods can aggravate symptoms and give discomfort.
The stomach has a greater number of parietal cells, and is hyperactive.	The stomach has fewer than normal parietal cells, and is often sluggish.
Mostly a male disorder.	About evenly divided between sexes.
Successful surgical treatment can be removal of the vagus nerve, *vagotomy*, or *selective vagotomy*.	Successful surgical treatment is usually removal of part of the stomach.

cause spasms of the adjacent muscles and swelling of surrounding tissue. This swelling can be an obstruction that can narrow the intestinal opening or close it off completely, preventing chyme from leaving the stomach and entering the intestines. In such cases, the victim can vomit the stomach contents, lose weight and develop other problems.

Recurrence of ulcers

Peptic ulcer disease is a chronic relapsing disorder. About 50 per cent of ulcer patients have another one within one or two years after the previous ulcer has healed. The longer period without a recurrence, the greater the likelihood that an ulcer will return.

When severe recurrent ulcers develop because of the production of several times the normal amounts of stomach acid, the condition is known as the Zollinger-Ellison Syndrome.

Ulcers and cancer

Many people worry that an ulcer may lead to cancer. Cancer of the duodenum is very rare so there is little chance of developing malignancy as a result of having a duodenal ulcer. However, with gastric ulcers the situation is less clear and a small percentage of stomach ulcers can be already malignant. Although there is little evidence that a peptic ulcer ever develops into cancer, there can be ulceration in a stomach cancer. And because stomach cancer can ulcerate or show some symptoms that are similar to those of a peptic ulcer, it is imperative to find out promptly whether the ulceration is truly a peptic ulcer or an ulcer with cancer. A determining factor used by a physician is often the amount of gastric acid produced: if you are making some acid, the ulcer is usually benign; the majority of patients with gastric cancer are incapable of producing acid.

What you can do
Check your diet to be sure you are having sensible meals, with attention to sufficient protein and vitamins. If acidic or spicy foods are bothersome, find out which ones cause distress, and avoid them.

A gradual increase in fibre may be beneficial, because fibrous foods need more chewing, and therefore more saliva, and saliva can buffer stomach acid.

Cut back on coffee, tea, cola drinks and chocolate; see the Caffeine section in Chapter 3 (page 36) for alternatives. Milk used to be a mainstay in the diets of ulcer patients, but it can have a 'rebound effect' and may actually be a potent stimulant of gastric acid secretion, with the fat, calcium and protein stimulating the production of even more acid. Doctors usually prohibit smoking by ulcer patients.

If you take non-prescription antacids, check Table 6 (page 83). Don't take antacids at the same time as certain other ulcer drugs, as they can interfere with absorption. Because of potential drug interactions if you are using antacids for a prolonged period, see your doctor before taking other medications.

Avoid using aspirin, whether plain or buffered; read labels of other non-prescription medicines as these compounds may also contain aspirin or salicylate. Your chemist or doctor can suggest alternatives without salicylate. Ulcer risk is smaller with enteric-coated aspirin which dissolves in the small intestine instead of the stomach. Consult your doctor about alternative drugs for arthritis and other chronic diseases.

Check stools regularly. See your doctor immediately if stools appear dark and tarry, or any rectal bleeding occurs, or if you vomit blood, have prolonged nausea or vomiting, or severe pain in your abdomen or back.

If you are vulnerable to stress at work, consider changing your job.

Doctors usually recommend that an ulcer patient should get plenty of sleep. In this way the body is rested, the stomach is at rest, and this can aid the healing process.

What the doctor can do
To determine treatment, the physician must first diagnose precisely the condition of the stomach and the position of the ulcer. The most common procedure to detect an ulcer is by barium X-ray. If an ulcer is not evident in an X-ray, the doctor uses a fibre-optic endoscope to view the inner surfaces of the digestive tract (gastroscopy). Analysis of stomach juices and biopsies of cells can determine the possibility of malignancy. The physician sometimes orders a second gastroscopy six to eight weeks after treatment to check that the ulcer has healed (an indication that it is benign), and be sure that no cancerous growth was missed.

The physician may prescribe histamine-blocking drugs such as *cimetidine* (Tagamet) or *ranitidine* (Zantac) (except during pregnancy) which are powerful inhibitors of stomach acid and pepsin secretion. These can relieve pain and promote ulcer healing within a few weeks, and may also be used for long-term therapy to prevent recurrent ulcers or if patients prefer not to have an operation. For short-term treatment (up to eight weeks) of duodenal ulcers, the drug *sucralfate* (Carafate) acts directly on the ulcer site by coating the ulcer and protecting the area from further acid damage. Anticholinergic drugs such as atropine, belladonna and the newer synthetics, are also used occasionally which decrease the action of the acid-producing cells, and change gastric motility.

Most ulcers heal successfully in response to these medications. But if an ulcer won't heal, the physician may decide on an operation, either removing the lower portion of the stomach (*antrectomy*) where gastrin is produced, or cutting the vagus nerve (*vagotomy*) which connects the brain to the stomach. A refined variation of this latter operation is called a *selective vagotomy* in which the procedure concentrates on cutting only those parts of the vagus nerve that go to the acid-secreting cells in the stomach wall.

Alternatively, the doctor may treat a bleeding ulcer by passing an electric current through the tissue to stop blood flow (*multipolar electrocoagulation*) or by using a heated aluminium cylinder (*heat probe*).

CHAPTER 9

The small intestine

Gallstones

The gallbladder's primary function is to store and secrete bile into the intestine at the proper time to aid in digestion. Bile is a yellowish fluid produced by the liver and is made up of soap-like chemicals that keep cholesterol in the gallbladder in liquid form. The gallbladder can store up to a cupful of bile.

Gallstones are clumps of solid material that form in the bile stored in the gallbladder. There are two major types: cholesterol stones and pigment stones.

Cholesterol stones are composed principally of cholesterol; pigment stones contain bile pigments such as bilirubin and other substances such as calcium. Stones can vary in size from a grain of sand to as big as an egg; the gallbladder may develop a single large stone or many smaller ones – even several thousand. Small stones can move into the bile ducts and become lodged, to block the flow of bile and causing pain and jaundice.

Gallstones form when certain chemicals in bile, either cholesterol or bile pigments, clump together. These clumps become the cores from which larger stones can grow. If more cholesterol or bile pigments are deposited, these masses can grow even larger – like an accumulating snowball rolling downhill.

Many people have gallstones but no symptoms. However, when gallbladder pain occurs, it is usually a steady, severe pain in the upper abdomen that may last as short as twenty or thirty minutes or as long as several hours. Pain may also be felt between the shoulder blades or in the right shoulder, and may cause nausea or vomiting.

If gallstones lodge in the common bile duct, they can block

bile flow not only from the gallbladder but also from the liver.
Stones may interfere with the flow of digestive fluids secreted by
the pancreas into the small intestine and lead to pancreatitis.

In rural areas of Africa, gallstones are almost nonexistent. The
highest incidence of gallstones in the United States occurs in
people of Mexican-American and Native American descent.
Among some American Indian tribes, such as the Pima Indians
of Arizona, 70 per cent of women have gallstones by the age of
30. The majority of American Indian men have gallstones by the
time they reach 60. American blacks of both sexes have the
lowest incidence of gallstones. White people in America have a
rate twice that of blacks. Although anyone may be a potential
candidate for gallstones, the condition occurs more often in
women than in men. People most likely to develop gallstones are

- women who have been pregnant, or who have used birth-
  control pills or menopausal oestrogen therapy;
- both men and women who are overweight;
- those over the age of 60;
- those who go on intensive slimming diets or who lose a lot of
  weight quickly.

What you can do
Maintain a sensible weight in relation to your height and frame.
Reduce consumption of fat and cholesterol in foods; increase
dietary fibre.

What the doctor can do
Diagnosis can be by X-rays, or by using an endoscope passed
through to the small intestine, or ultrasound equipment which
avoids exposure to radiation.

The most common method for treating gallstones is the
removal of the gallbladder, then a search in the bile ducts for any
stones that may have passed into these channels. Removal of the
gallbladder does not seem to affect the digestion process. Non-
surgical treatments include using an endoscope to widen the
bile duct, which does not remove stones but allows them to pass
harmlessly into the intestinal tract. When a patient has multiple
small cholesterol-containing stones, and a few acute symptoms,
the stones may be dissolved chemically by using drugs such as

Ursodiol, Monooctanoin (Moctanin) or Chenodiol (Chenix), although this treatment may take one or two years to work. Shock-wave therapy, *lithotripsy*, (developed in West Germany as a method of shattering kidney stones instead of removing them through surgery) is being tested on gallstones, when a patient has larger but fewer stones.

Gallbladder disease

The term *porcelain gallbladder* is used to describe a condition where the gallbladder itself is calcified, rather than merely containing stones. The gallbladder cannot function properly which this happens because the walls of the sac can no longer contract. Removal of the organ is necessary. If left untreated, there is a greatly increased risk of gallbladder cancer, which is serious because it starts without many symptoms and spreads rapidly.

Pancreatitis

Behind the stomach is the large gland called the pancreas producing digestive secretions that normally empty into the small intestine through a duct. Inflammation of the pancreas (*pancreatitis*) is thought to occur when digestive enzymes attack the pancreatic tissues, leading to damage of the gland. Severe cases can be accompanied by bleeding into the gland, further gland destruction and the formation of cysts or abscesses. If the pancreas is not permanently damaged, the condition is referred to as *acute* pancreatitis, whereas when permanent damage to the pancreas takes place, it is called *chronic*.

Acute pancreatitis is usually caused by the abuse of alcohol, or by gallstones, abdominal surgery and trauma, certain drugs, cancer and pregnancy. The disease may also, on rare occasions, result from infections such as mumps. Symptoms usually begin with a mild steady pain in the upper abdomen becoming increasingly severe, lasting for several days. The abdomen may be swollen and extremely tender, and it is sometimes possible to feel a lump in the area. Other symptoms may include nausea, vomiting, low-grade fever, increased pulse rate and jaundice. People with acute pancreatitis develop metabolic disturbances, such as elevated blood sugar and blood lipids (fats). The acute form rarely progresses to chronic pancreatitis, but some people may already have permanent damage to the gland caused by alcohol.

Chronic pancreatitis is usually caused by alcoholism; heredity, diet and other diseases may also contribute. It is more common in men than women, and usually develops between the ages of 30 and 50. Symptoms are abdominal pain, and later weight loss and diarrhoea. Poor digestion may lead to *steatorrhoea* (increasing amounts of fat in stools). Diabetes may also develop at this stage.

What you can do
Cut down on drinking alcohol, reduce consumption of fatty foods, and don't overeat.

What the doctor can do
Surgery is sometimes required to help in the diagnosis and treatment of acute pancreatitis, when there are complications such as an abscess, cyst or bleeding. When gallstones are found, they are usually removed. Treatment of chronic pancreatitis is directed at the relief of pain and the management of disturbances of metabolism. Dietary fats are restricted, and supplementary pancreatic enzymes may be provided to reduce the amount of fat lost in stools. Occasionally, insulin must be given to control blood sugar. In rare cases, surgery is needed if there is a narrowing of the pancreatic duct or common bile duct. Occasionally, part or all of the pancreas will be removed in an attempt to relieve chronic pain. Most patients with alcoholic pancreatitis can prevent recurrent attacks by total abstinence from alcohol. Even when the pancreas is permanently damaged, there can be improvement in absorption and nutrition if no alcohol is consumed.

Cancer of the pancreas

Pancreatic cancer is often advanced before it is detected, because of the hidden location of the pancreas and a variety of symptoms that can also be the symptoms of other diseases. It usually causes jaundice, intense itching of the skin, abdominal pain and discomfort, nausea, diarrhoea, belching, a feeling of fullness and intolerance of fatty foods. Other symptoms include weight loss, loss of appetite and loss of energy.

What the doctor can do
Your physician can determine more clearly where the tumour is situated by using barium X-rays, liver-function studies, angiography, and a biopsy test of tissue. There are two kinds of cancer of the pancreas: *islet-cell carcinoma* of the *endocrine* pancreas and *adenocarcinoma* of the *exocrine* pancreas. Cancer of the endocrine pancreas is highly treatable and often curable. Cancer of the exocrine pancreas, on the other hand, is more difficult to treat and not often curable. In some cases, the physician will remove a part of or the entire pancreas. When the pancreas is entirely removed, medicines are prescribed to substitute for its function, and the patient is put on a permanent low-sugar low-fat diet with supplementary vitamin K.

Some conditions of the liver

Hepatitis

Inflammation of the liver may be caused by viruses, poisons, drugs or alcohol.

Viral hepatitis can take several forms:

Type A hepatitis (formerly known as infectious hepatitis), is caused by a virus that enters via the mouth, spread by personal contact with infected people, and by faecally-contaminated food and water. Symptoms can be so mild that you may not be aware of its presence, although it can still be passed on to others. They are similar to those for flu or gastroenteritis in the beginning, including nausea, abdominal discomfort, fever and headache, and a tenderness in the liver area (upper right side of the abdomen). Urine may be dark. After four to seven days, jaundice may develop, along with nausea, vomiting and light-coloured stools.

Type B hepatitis (formerly known as serum hepatitis), and the recently-detected Type C, are caused by viruses found in all body fluids of infected persons, including blood, semen, saliva and urine, rather than in faeces. They are spread by intimate contact with infected people, contaminated blood transfusions, or when contaminated needles are shared by drug addicts or used in medical or dental procedures. Next to alcohol abuse, hepatitis B is probably the major cause of cirrhosis of the liver and liver cancer. The symptoms are much the same as for Type A, with the difference being an outbreak of itching red weals (hives) early in the course of the disease. At highest risk of acquiring Type B and Type C infections are dialysis patients, haemophiliacs who receive blood products frequently, those who inject themselves with illicit drugs, dentists and dental hygienists, physicians, nursing staff, medical students, and laboratory technicians handling blood or urine samples.

Type C hepatitis (previously known as non-A, non-B) is infection caused by one or more viruses that cannot be traced to Type A, B or D hepatitis viruses, and is a risk for anyone who must receive transfused blood or blood products.

Type D hepatitis (also known as delta hepatitis), is an infection that exists only in combination with hepatitis B virus, to produce a disease more severe than Type B alone. People with a hepatitis B infection, or those who are carriers of Type B virus, are at risk of acquiring hepatitis D. Type D is spread in the same ways as hepatitis B. High risk people are dialysis patients, haemophiliacs who receive blood products frequently, or those who inject illicit drugs.

What you can do
Be sure food and water supplies are clean and free of contamination. Wash hands after using the toilet. Don't take illicit drugs. Avoid unnecessary piercing of the skin such as acupuncture, ear-piercing or tattooing when instruments may be contaminated and pose a serious risk of passing hepatitis to others. Vaccination is recommended for highest-risk medical personnel. If you do contract hepatitis, bed rest is advisable when symptoms are at their height. Have a well-balanced diet, with sufficient calories to avoid malnutrition.

What the doctor can do
He or she can give a simple blood test to determine with

certainty if you have hepatitis. Some doctors give injections of immune serum globulin to families of hepatitis patients.

Toxic hepatitis is a serious liver inflammation caused by some drugs, and chemicals used in certain occupations such as dry-cleaning fluids (carbon tetrachloride), insecticides, industrial solvents and various metallic compounds. Drugs causing liver damage may be sulpha drugs, potent tranquillizers (such as chlorpromazine), bromates and some antibiotics. Symptoms include nausea, vomiting, diarrhoea, collapse, usually followed by jaundice.

What you can do
Prevent accidental ingestion by handling chemicals carefully. Check the lead content of your drinking water with the water company. Consult your doctor about the correct dosage and effect of the medicines you have been prescribed.

Alcoholic liver disease

This is a term that includes several ailments: *fatty liver* denotes an excess of fat deposits; *alcoholic hepatitis* is caused by the abuse of alcohol, and is marked by inflammation of the liver with cells dying; *cirrhosis* is when the liver is badly scarred or swollen, and the formation of scars on liver tissue is sufficiently severe to cause dysfunction. It may be caused by severe hepatitis, by heavy drinking, or by drugs as with toxic hepatitis. The majority of cases of cirrhosis are due to chronic alcoholism. However, in those parts of the world where viral hepatitis is common, cirrhosis is mainly caused by hepatitis. Cirrhosis may not cause symptoms until the disease is far advanced.

What you can do
Cut out drinking alcohol. Reduce fatty foods in your diet.

Cancer of the liver

This cancer is a common problem among alcoholics. The risk of this disease is increased when the liver is constantly overloaded with a buildup of unused fatty acids. Fats increase the production of bile acids, and some bile acids have been observed to act as promoters of tumour growth. The consumption of certain seeds with a high oil content, such as peanuts, is linked to cancers of the liver, apparently because of a particular fungus, *Aspergillus flavus*, which is a parasite of oily seeds.

Secondary liver cancer is a result of the spread of cancer from elsewhere in the body (frequently the breast or colon), not cured by surgery or other treatment.

Symptoms of liver cancer are not obvious, although in later stages there may be weight loss, loss of appetite, and possibly fever and jaundice.

What you can do
Cut out drinking alcohol. Reduce consumption of fats in your diet.

What the doctor can do
Tumours of the liver may be malignant or benign. Benign tumours are small, produce no symptoms and are usually discovered only during the course of another operation. The doctor may make a diagnosis using radiography, endoscopy, liver scans, and biopsy tests of liver tissue. If cancer is confined to a segment or lobe in the liver, surgical removal is usually performed. If cancer has spread to other parts of the body, extensive surgery may be too debilitating.

Appendicitis

The appendix becomes inflamed or infected when the opening between the caecum and the appendix is blocked. Appendicitis is related to a diet that is low in fibre. Low-fibre foods produce smaller harder stools. Pieces of stool, called *faecaliths* (literally stones made of faeces), can obstruct the opening of the appendix, or the blockage may occur with a small fruit pip.

As appendicitis begins, the blocked organ becomes distended and nausea may progress to vomiting. Typical pain starts around the navel (not even close to where the appendix lies). With still further swelling of the appendix, veins become blocked off, blood stagnates within the appendix, and bacteria multiply when they are no longer carried away in the blood. As the wall of the appendix becomes infected, it inflames the peritoneum of the abdominal wall which it touches, producing severe pain in the right lower quadrant, below the navel and on the right side.

What you can do
Have well-balanced meals that have enough fibre for your
system. If symptoms of appendicitis occur, medical help should
be sought *without delay*. Don't wait for the appendix to perforate,
and risk having *peritonitis*.

If you are away from civilization, what can you do? In an
emergency when medical help is not available, put yourself in
Fowler's position. (This procedure is *not* a substitute for surgery,
but only a control of the condition until expert surgery is
available.) It is a semi-sitting position, with your back up at least
45 degrees from horizontal, and with a blanket or pillow under
the knees to avoid stretching abdominal muscles. Take no
cathartic, enema, food or drink. In the Fowler position, you help
assure that, should the appendix perforate, pus will settle by
gravity into the lowest part of the abdomen, and give a better
chance for an abscess to form and wall off the infection, preventing it from spreading through the abdomen.

Once nausea has passed, sip small amounts of water throughout the day, or sip tea or a clear broth. Do not drink full-strength
fruit juices or coffee which may stimulate bowel contraction. If
fever should develop, take aspirin or acetaminophen. A cold
pack over the abdomen can be helpful in diminishing pain.

What the doctor can do
Removal of an appendix today is usually a relatively simple
procedure that takes half an hour or less. The patient is usually
up the next day, and eating a normal diet within a few days.

CHAPTER 10

The lower tract

Although it is relatively short – only a fifth of the total length of the intestinal tract – the colon is the site of a surprising variety of unpleasant and sometimes life-threatening disorders. Virtually no part of this organ is immune from disease, ranging from appendicitis at the point where the colon begins to haemorrhoids at the point where it ends. In between, the colon is beset by inflammatory and infectious diseases, including inflammatory bowel disease, diverticulosis, irritable bowel syndrome, intestinal polyps and, of course, cancers. The intestines (sometimes called the bowel) can be injured in many different ways. The bowel may be infected by a wide variety of viruses, bacteria, or parasites that produce diarrhoea; other disturbances cause constipation. It may be damaged by chemical poisoning, radiation exposure, surgery, physical injury or disturbances of its blood supply, any of which may cause acute or chronic inflammation of long duration – for months, years, or a lifetime.

One common trouble is flatulence – which is usually more of a social than a medical problem.

Flatulence

The subject of wind and flatulence is probably an embarrassing one for most people, and not one that we talk about. But the truth is that we all naturally have gas in our intestinal tract and release it one way or another.

How much wind does the body normally produce? It varies considerably from person to person. Most of us produce somewhere between 400 to 2,400cc of *flatus* each day. Studies show that in some people even as little as 30 to 200cc of gas in the intestine can cause spasms of the bowel after eating.

The principal component of flatus is *nitrogen* which comes from swallowed air. When undigested bits of food, such as bran or lactose, enter the colon, bacteria ferment the particles, producing *carbon dioxide, hydrogen* and other gases, usually in a small amount. Some people also produce *methane*, though its production does not seem to be affected by diet. The major components of flatus are odourless; any unpleasant odour is caused by trace gases such as *hydrogen sulphide*.

What causes wind? Each time you swallow, small amounts of air enter the stomach. Increased amounts from air-swallowing can occur if you have nervous tension or poorly-fitting dentures, if you sip very hot drinks slowly, drink carbonated beverages such as beer, champagne, effervescent bottled water or fizzy soft drinks, if you chew gum, or have postnasal drip. Gas in the stomach may accumulate to be belched out, or it may pass into the small intestine where part of it is absorbed. The gas that is diffused through the intestinal wall into the blood gets carried to the lungs and exhaled in the breath as a waste product. The rest travels into the colon to be passed out through the rectum.

The foods you eat can be a factor in the production of gas. Some foods such as cooked dried beans, cauliflower, brussels sprouts, broccoli, cabbage and bran are not completely digested in the small intestine. When the undigested pieces of food reach the colon, they arrive in a form that the body cannot absorb (mainly cellulose, and *oligosaccharides* – sugars with up to five molecules). So the large population of colon bacteria goes to work on them with fermentation, and this fermentation process often gives off various gases (primarily carbon dioxide) as waste products. This is a normal process.

Although fibre plays a useful role in good nutrition and health, a rapid increase of fibre intake can result in some distressing side effects. If you are unaccustomed to eating more whole unpro-cessed bran, or more wholegrain cereals and breads, these can leave you feeling stuffed or bloated. The digestive system works best if it is allowed to adjust slowly to any dietary change, and while it is adapting to handling an increase in fibre, your digestive system may well produce more gas.

Excess gas can also be caused by lactase enzyme deficiency.

When lactose (the sugar found in milk and other dairy products) passes undigested into the colon because of insufficient lactase enzyme, bacteria ferment the sugar, creating gas. See the section on lactose intolerance in Chapter 3.

Another possible source of intestinal gas may be carbon dioxide: when stomach acid enters the duodenum, it is neutralized by bicarbonate. Carbon dioxide is released during this process. Most of the gas is absorbed into the blood. What the remaining carbon dioxide does is unclear, but some scientists believe it may play a role in producing gaseous symptoms.

Some people can dispel upper abdominal pressure and pain by belching after eating. But gas can collect anywhere in the colon and can lead to pain and bloating. When it accumulates on the right side of the colon, the pain can be similar to that caused by gallbladder disease. Gas in the upper left portion of the colon can result in a condition called the *splenic flexure syndrome*. The pain associated with this condition can spread to the left side of the chest and be confused with heart disease.

A feeling of distension of the abdomen is a common complaint. It often increases during the day and is most severe after the largest meal. Distension occurs more often in women who have had one or more pregnancies, or in people who have lost the tone of their abdominal rectus muscles due to age or disease. If your abdomen is distended when you sit or stand, but not when you are lying down, the distension is probably related to muscular weakness rather than excess gas. A support garment, or exercise to increase rectus muscle tone such as sit-ups may relieve symptoms.

If the frequency, odour or volume is excessive and troublesome, it is possible that your symptoms are the result of a 'functional disorder' where there are no signs of disease and yet your intestinal tract sometimes does not seem to function properly. A functional disorder may cause discomfort, but it is not serious and does not lead to a serious disease. Recent research suggests a possible explanation: the digestive tract seems to be governed by a delicate pattern of electrical impulses, in much the same way that the muscles of the heart are governed. Some researchers think that when these electrical impulses are disrupted, the contractions of the intestinal muscles become disorganized. This disorganization can result in a variety of symptoms, including pain, diarrhoea, constipation, bloating, and a sensation that there is too much gas in the system.

What you can do

Eat meals slowly and chew food thoroughly; don't sip beverages when they are too hot. Avoid chewing gum or sucking boiled sweets. Eliminate from your diet such carbonated beverages as beer and soft drinks. Eat fewer gas-producing foods such as cauliflower, brussels sprouts, beans, broccoli, cabbage and bran, until your system can accommodate them comfortably. If lactase deficiency is causing gas, you need to cut back on dairy foods. If abdominal bloating is your problem, try exercises such as sit-ups to increase muscle tone. Check with your dentist to make sure dentures fit properly.

Some people believe that antacids can be used to relieve gas pains but this is not so. Antacids may be helpful for heartburn and peptic ulcers, but they do not relieve symptoms attributed to gas.

In the end, flatulence is more of a social embarrassment than a medical problem – if it doesn't bother you, don't worry about it. But when belching or flatulence is persistent and troublesome in its frequency, you should seek medical attention.

What the doctor can do

Your physician may simply prescribe simethicone, or want to perform tests to ensure that your symptoms are not caused by abnormalities such as enzyme deficiencies in your digestive tract.

Activated charcoal can soak up gas until it is secreted in stool, but discuss this first with your doctor as charcoal can also soak up any other medicine you may take and block its effectiveness.

Constipation

Frequency of bowel movements among normal, healthy people varies greatly – thrice daily to thrice weekly. Perfectly healthy people may fall outside both ends of this range. As a rule, however, if more than three days pass without a bowel movement, the intestinal contents may harden and you may have difficulty or even pain during elimination. Stool may harden and be painful to pass even after shorter intervals between bowel movements.

There are many common misconceptions and false beliefs concerning 'proper' bowel habits and what constitutes constipation. The word 'regularity' has been in our vocabulary for over 200 years as a genteel way to refer to a timely bowel movement, but how regular is regular? One person's constipation can be another's definition of regularity. One fallacy about bowel regularity is that you must have a bowel movement every day in order to be 'normal'. This is absolutely incorrect. Good health does *not* require the bowels to perform like clockwork. Another common misconception is that wastes stored in the body are absorbed and are dangerous to health or shorten the life span.

Such fears and fallacies have led to a marked overuse and abuse of laxatives. Many people have become conditioned or brainwashed by advertising that perpetuates the once-a-day idea that equates good health with clockwork daily bowel movements. Millions of pounds are spent every year on laxatives; many are unnecessary and some are harmful. The use of all laxatives should be minimized, because they can be habit-forming and have the potential for causing diarrhoea. See Table 8 for a review of typical non-prescription laxatives.

TABLE 8

REVIEW OF TYPICAL NON-PRESCRIPTION LAXATIVES

Laxative type	How it works	How quickly?	Ingredients
Bulk forming	Increases the volume and water content of stool, makes it softer and promotes bowel movement.	In 12 to 72 hours.	Bran, methyl-cellulose, karaya, malt soup extract, polycarbophil, psyllium seeds or husks.
Hyperosmotic	Attracts water into the stool.	In 15 minutes to 1 hour.	Glycerin, sorbitol.

Laxative type	How it works	How quickly?	Ingredients
Lubricant	Lubricates the contents of the intestinal tract to soften stool and make it slip more easily down the intestine.	Oral form: 6 to 8 hours. Rectal form: 2 to 15 minutes.	Liquid paraffin (mineral oil).
Saline	Increases water in the intestine.	Oral form: 30 minutes to 6 hours. Rectal form: 2 to 15 minutes.	Magnesium citrate, magnesium hydroxide, magnesium sulphate, sodium phosphate, sodium biphosphate.
Stimulant	Causes rhythmic contractions of the small or large intestine.	Oral form: 6 to 12 hours. Rectal form: 15 minutes to 1 hour.	Aloe, bisacodyl, casanthranol, cascara, castor oil, danthron, dehydrocholic acid, phenolphthalein, senna.
Stool softener	Penetrates stool, providing it with moisture to soften.	Oral form: 12 to 72 hours. Rectal form: 2 to 15 minutes.	Docusate salts (causes birth defects in animals).
Carbon-dioxide releasing suppository	Releases carbon dioxide inducing gentle pressure in the rectum.	5 to 30 minutes.	Combination of sodium biphosphate, anhydrous sodium acid pyrophosphate and sodium bicarbonate; and a combination of sodium bisphosphate and sodium bitartrate.

Constipation is not a disease but a symptom. Most people experience an occasional brief bout of constipation, an interruption of routine that is minor and temporary, and which corrects itself with diet and time. However, chronic constipation can be caused by many different conditions, of which the most common are:

Imaginary constipation. This results from misconceptions about what is 'normal' and what is not. In their slavery to the clock or calendar, some people abuse laxatives, suppositories and enemas. This type of constipation can be 'cured' by giving reassurance that their frequency of bowel movement *is* normal.

Irritable Bowel Syndrome. Some people develop spasms of the colon which delay the speed at which the contents of the intestine move through the digestive tract.

Bad bowel habits. Ignoring the urge to defecate, some people are 'too busy', or want to avoid using public toilets. After a while, a person may stop feeling the urge, which leads to progressive constipation.

Poor diet. Meals that are high in animal fats (meats, dairy products, eggs), refined sugar and refined flours (rich desserts and other sweets), but low in fibre and low in liquids. There is no fibre in meat, fish, fats, sugar, milk or alcoholic drinks; insufficient roughage discourages peristaltic contractions.

Lack of exercise. People who are bedridden, confined to wheelchairs or elderly persons who are housebound, are often subject to sluggish bowels and the weakness that result from muscular inactivity.

Laxative abuse. If you habitually take laxatives, you become dependent on them and require increased dosages. Finally the intestine becomes insensitive and fails to work properly. Over-reliance on bowel-movement aids can also bring about diarrhoea or real constipation by inducing 'lazy bowel syndrome'.

Travel. People often experience constipation when travelling. This may relate to changes in lifestyle, diet, drinking insufficient water, not allowing enough time, unfamiliar toilets, or not responding promptly to the urge to defecate.

Pregnancy. Constipation may be due partly to the pressure of the growing foetus compressing the intestine, partly to hormonal changes in the glands during pregnancy, or drinking more milk or taking calcium supplements.

Medications. A large number of medicines can cause constipation, including pain medications (especially narcotics), antacids containing aluminium or calcium, antispasmodic drugs, antidepressant drugs, tranquillizers, anticonvulsants for epilepsy, calcium supplements and iron supplements. On the other hand, taking laxatives may interfere with the effectiveness of other medicines you need to use.

Fissures and Haemorrhoids. Painful conditions of the anus can produce a spasm of the anal sphincter, which aggravates constipation.

Hormonal or Gland Disturbances. Certain hormonal fluctuations and disturbances such as an underactive thyroid gland, can produce constipation.

Mechanical Compression. Scarring, inflammation around diverticula, tumours, and cancer can produce compression of the intestines.

Nerve Damage. Injuries to the spinal cord and tumours pressing on the spinal cord may produce constipation by affecting the nerves that lead to the intestine.

Loss of Body Salts. Loss of body salts through the kidneys, or through vomiting or diarrhoea, can be a cause.

Other diseases. Diseases that affect the body tissues such as scleroderma or lupus, and other conditions such as multiple sclerosis, Parkinson's disease and stroke, or gynaecological operations such as hysterectomy can be responsible for constipation.

Constipation is a common problem in children, and may be related to any of the causes previously noted. But in a small number of children, constipation may be a symptom of physical problems: children with such defects as the absence of normal nerve endings in portions of the bowel, abnormalities of the spinal cord, thyroid deficiency, mental retardation, and certain other inherited metabolic disorders.

Many children who suffer from constipation when they are older have a history of passing stools that are firmer than average in their early weeks of life. Constipation may result in pain when the child has bowel movements. Also cracks in the skin (fissures) may develop in the anus and these fissures can bleed or increase pain, making a child withhold stools.

Most children's constipation, however, is due to poor bowel habits. Some children withhold stools because they dislike school toilets or other toilets away from home. Or withholding may be made worse because of severe emotional problems caused by stress from family crises or difficulties with schoolwork.

If periods between bowel movements become quite long – longer than one or two weeks – children may develop faecal impactions where the stool is packed so tightly in the bowel that the normal expelling action of the bowel is unable to evacuate the stool, making it impossible to pass spontaneously.

The elderly are five times more likely than young people to have problems with constipation. Constipation is often the result of poor diet (because of a low budget or poor teeth), insufficient intake of liquids, lack of exercise, the use of certain drugs to treat other conditions, and poor bowel habits. In addition, experts agree that too often older people become too concerned with having a bowel movement, and that constipation is frequently an imaginary ailment.

Many older persons who are single or widowed may have a lack of interest in eating, and may rely heavily on convenience foods, and foods which are low in fibre; older people may have lost their natural teeth or have problems with dentures and may choose soft processed foods which tend to be lacking in 'bulk'. They sometimes cut back on liquids, especially if they are not eating regular or balanced meals, whereas water and other fluids add bulk to stools, making bowel movements softer and easier to pass.

Lack of exercise may contribute to constipation in the elderly, especially if prolonged bed rest is necessary after an accident or during an illness. Many elderly persons need drugs prescribed for other conditions, for example certain antidepressants, antacids containing aluminium or calcium, antihistamines, diuretics and anti-Parkinsonism drugs, and these can produce constipation in some people.

When older people (or younger persons such as bulimics) become preoccupied with bowel movements, this can lead them to depend heavily on habit-forming laxatives. When the bowel begins to rely on laxatives or becomes used to enemas, the natural mechanisms fail to work without the help of drugs, leading to loss of normal function.

The use and misuse of enemas

The use of enemas is limited. Too many enemas, like too many laxatives, can lead to a dependence on such products. An enema can serve a useful purpose under the right circumstances, when for instance patients are being prepared for surgery, X-ray examinations or child delivery. But some people overuse enemas to maintain 'regularity'. Even if only water is used, frequent enemas can deplete the body of essential minerals.

Homemade enemas sometimes contain soapsuds to help move impacted faeces, but they have been known to cause acute inflammatory reactions in the colon within hours of their use. More serious problems from soapsuds enemas can be rectal gangrene, acute haemorrhagic colitis, kidney failure and even death.

Colonic irrigation or the high colonic enema is another type of enema not recommended by doctors. It really does go too far in the literal sense. A high colonic enema involves passing a rubber tube into the colon, via the rectum, for a distance of about 75cm (30 inches), whereas an ordinary enema tube is only 7.5cm (3 inches) long. Warm water is pumped in and then out, a few pints at a time, using up to 75 litres (20 gallons) before the procedure is completed. Coffee, herbs, enzymes, wheat, and grass extract are often added to the mix, sometimes administered as often as every two hours. Colonic irrigation is alleged to remove poisons and rot that are supposed to accumulate in the gut, purifying the whole body as well as the colon. But there is *no* scientific evidence that colonic irrigation will do any of these things. The procedure can be dangerous. Repeated coffee enemas have resulted in deaths from electrolyte imbalance, bowel perforation, death of bowel tissue (gangrene) and toxic colitis.

Constipation itself is usually not serious, but it may be a signal and the only noticeable symptom of an underlying serious disease of the colon, or even cancer. Also constipation itself can lead to complications such as *haemorrhoids* caused by extreme straining, or *fissures* in the anal opening, caused by the hard stool stretching the sphincters. *Bleeding* can occur from either of these two sources and appear as bright red streaks on the surface of the stool. Fissures may be quite painful and can aggravate the constipation that originally caused them. Faecal *impactions* tend to occur in the very young and in the elderly, and may be accompanied by a loss of control of stool, with liquid stool flowing around the hard impaction. Occasionally, straining causes a small amount of intestinal lining to push out from the rectal opening. This is known as a *rectal prolapse*, and may lead to secretion of mucus. In children, this may be a feature of cystic fibrosis.

What you can do

Prevention is the best treatment. Rely less on laxative medications, suppositories and enemas, and more on high-fibre foods to prevent or relieve constipation. Know what is normal for *you*. In this way you can avoid developing a laxative habit by treating constipation that does not really exist. Here are five steps to help you avoid constipation:

1. Eat a well-balanced diet with an increased amount of fibrous foods including unprocessed bran, wholegrain breads and wholegrain cereals, prunes and prune juice, fresh unpeeled fruits, seed-filled berries and vegetables. See Table 3 on page 35 for examples.
2. Drink plenty of liquids: a glass of hot water when you rise in the morning, and a glass about 30 minutes before each meal. Water, juices and other fluids help promote bowel action (but milk and milk products can be constipating).
3. Exercise regularly – a brisk walk, cycling, swimming – whatever you can manage comfortably. Special exercises such as curl-ups can be helpful to tone up abdominal muscles after pregnancy or if muscles used in defecation are weak.
4. Set aside plenty of time after breakfast or dinner to allow for undisturbed visits to the toilet.
5. Never ignore the urge to defecate.

The importance of fibre in maintaining normal elimination has been recognized for centuries, but recently there has been renewed interest. Researchers have reported that high-fibre intake not only helps relieve constipation but also reduces the incidence of gallstones, diverticulosis, irritable colon and haemorrhoids.

Fibre in foods can be *water-soluble* or *water-insoluble*; it's good to have some of both.

Water-soluble fibre has gums and pectins which dissolve with body fluids to form gel-like substances effective for increasing bulk and promoting laxation, for reducing the body's absorption of fat, lowering blood cholesterol and triglycerides, reducing risk of cancers of the colon and rectum, and losing weight. It can moderate blood sugars and improve mineral absorption. Examples: oatbran, oatmeal, dried beans, dried peas, apples (including skins) and citrus fruits.

On the other hand, *water-insoluble* fibre cannot be dissolved in water nor broken down by digestive enzymes, but it can absorb water, swell up and add bulk. It protects against digestive tract problems. It keeps food moving along, improves peristaltic contractions, remedies constipation, reduces risk of colon cancers, decreases risk of diverticulosis, and helps with weight loss – but too much may cause mineral loss. Examples: whole grains, wheatbran, and wholewheat breads and breakfast cereals. (Note that some breads are merely dark with caramel colouring and not wholemeal flour.)

Since insoluble fibre holds water, stools produced by a high-fibre diet tend to be bulkier and softer and pass more quickly and more easily through the intestines. This puts less strain and pressure on the bowel and blood vessels. Toxic substances that may be present in food, such as carcinogens, stay in the body for a shorter time.

If you do have a laxative habit, substitute milder ones, then gradually withdraw altogether, while improving your diet.

You may be constipated if more than three days pass between bowel movements, or if you have difficulty or pain passing a hardened stool; after all, most people experience constipation occasionally. However, if it becomes necessary to take laxatives or suppositories, do not use them for longer than two or three weeks without the advice of your doctor.

People on low-salt diets should not use laxative products containing sodium, unless directed by a doctor. Milk of Magnesia is a satisfactory laxative, but may overload the system with magnesium and should not be used if you have pain in the abdomen, since it could cause perforation of an acute appendix or rupture of a blocked bowel, if either condition should be present. Liquid paraffin (mineral oil) coats the intestine with an oily barrier; overuse may reduce the absorption of vitamins A,

D, E, and K, and can cause embarrassment by dripping from the anus unexpectedly. Liquid paraffin may also interact with some drugs, causing undesirable side effects.

Consult your doctor if you have abdominal pain of unknown cause, need a laxative for longer than three weeks, fail to have a bowel movement after using a laxative, have inflammatory bowel disorders, or a significant and prolonged change in your usual bowel habits, serious haemorrhoids, fissures, rectal bleeding, faecal impaction or obstruction.

Constipation in infants is often a signal of some more serious condition. As a general rule, non-prescription laxatives should not be given to children under two, lubricant laxatives should not be given to children under six, enteric-coated stimulant laxatives should not be used by children under six, and oral dosage forms of laxatives containing phosphates should not be given to children under five.

What the doctor can do
Your physician can prescribe special laxatives to relieve weakened patients who have to strain to move their bowels.

A doctor can determine if constipation is the symptom of an underlying disorder such as abnormalities or obstructions. In addition to routine blood, urine and stool tests, he may use a barium X-ray, a proctoscope or colonoscope to detect problems in the rectum, lower colon and intestine. If an underactive thyroid is causing constipation, thyroid extract may be prescribed.

Diarrhoea

If you dose yourself with too much bran or laxative to cure constipation, you may over-succeed and suffer the opposite problem: diarrhoea. This is when the large intestine pushes food through too quickly, perhaps because infections are irritating the intestine, so little fluid has a chance to be absorbed and the faeces are watery. Diarrhoea can be extremely debilitating because it represents a loss of important body fluids, water and minerals. In the case of small children, who have a very small reserve of water, unchecked diarrhoea can easily be fatal.

What is diarrhoea? The change from the general pattern of stools to frequent watery bowel movements is usually referred to as diarrhoea. As a rule, symptoms disappear after one or two days, and the only important effect is that water and salts are lost from the body. For most people, the short-lived episode is more of an inconvenience than an illness. But sometimes diarrhoea lasts for weeks or months, and then it can be an indication of major disease. This more serious form of diarrhoea may have blood, mucus, or undigested food in the stools. The disease that is causing diarrhoea may also produce fever, abdominal cramps, weight loss, nausea and/or vomiting.

What causes diarrhoea? It can be a symptom of a hundred or more different conditions or diseases. It can be brought on by excessive alcohol, overindulging in rich food, or caused by an emotional upset. The most common form is the one caused by a simple infection of a virus, by parasites, absorption defects such as lactose intolerance, nervousness, some drugs in certain cases, excessive amounts of sorbitol (an artificial sweetener) or post-operative conditions such as after removal of the gall-bladder. Aged persons may have a form of diarrhoea related to bacteria from the colon invading the small intestine, disrupting normal digestion. The elderly may also have faecal incontinence due to weakened anal sphincter muscles.

'Nervous diarrhoea' is part of the irritable bowel syndrome, and is very common during times of personal stress. However, some people suffer nervous stress fairly constantly, and may have continuous diarrhoea because of this.

'Intestinal flu' is often due to one of a number of viruses that infect the bowel, making it weep fluid; the excess of fluid in the bowel leads to liquid stools. The inflammation may also be associated with cramping abdominal pain, nausea and vomiting.

'Travellers' diarrhoea' is due to a particular bacteria common in certain areas of the world. People living in these areas are usually well-adjusted to the bacteria, although simple infectious diarrhoea is still a major killer in underdeveloped countries, where infections of the bowel are estimated to cause millions of deaths annually among infants. Travellers arriving in these areas are susceptible to these bacterial infections. Contaminated food or water, public swimming pools, and communal hot tubs are possible sources of these infections. See the Travel section in Chapter 4 (page 61).

Watery stools also contain salt, and severe diarrhoea causes the body to lose large amounts of water and salt. Since diarrhoea is often accompanied by vomiting, and you cannot keep solid food down, dietary intake is seriously reduced. Dangerous dehydration can occur in people poorly prepared to take these losses of fluid and salt, and it is especially critical in very young children, the elderly or people already weakened by major illness.

Fortunately most of the severe causes are rare. They include ulcerative colitis (when blood is usually present in stools), Crohn's disease, some forms of intestinal cancer (when pain and weight loss might also be present), and some disorders of the intestine that lead to poor digestion of food.

What you can do

Anybody with diarrhoea should drink plenty of fluids – safe bottled water and tinned fruit juices – and have complete rest in bed. See the doctor as soon as possible if there is still vomiting or diarrhoea after 12 to 24 hours, especially if the person is very young, old, or otherwise weak. A thorough medical examination is needed.

Some kinds of infectious diarrhoea may be followed by temporary malabsorption, which means that after the infection subsides, the digestive system will not tolerate large amounts of milk, dairy products, or foods high in fat for one to three weeks. Temporary malabsorption causes symptoms similar to infectious diarrhoea – cramping, nausea, vomiting and diarrhoea. Such sensitivity may be reduced by drinking sweet acidophilus milk.

What the doctor can do

An examination of stools and urine is usually required for the growth of organisms by culture, or a blood test for antibodies. Infections with salmonella (such as typhoid fever), shigella (dysentery), amoebae, and some other organisms may require specific treatment such as antibiotics, although these may not be automatically prescribed because of undesirable side effects. Some drugs, such as entero-vioform, that were used for diarrhoea in the past, are now considered dangerous.

Food poisoning

Most food poisoning involves the gastrointestinal tract. A notable exception is botulism which attacks the nervous system, causing progressive paralysis of the respiratory system, and making breathing, swallowing and speaking difficult.

Although the symptoms of food poisoning are all somewhat similar, the organisms (or their by-products) that cause the illness are varied. They include bacteria, bacterial toxins, viruses, mycotoxins from moulds, and protozoa (one-celled microscopic parasites). Most of them cannot be seen, smelled or tasted. The leading trouble-makers are:

Campylobacter jejuni bacteria from untreated water, raw or undercooked meat, poulty or shellfish, and unpasteurized milk. Symptoms: severe (possibly bloody) diarrhoea, cramping, fever and headache.

Clostridium botulinum bacteria, producing botulism, from home-canned or other canned foods. Symptoms: double vision, droopy eyelids, difficulty in speaking, swallowing or breathing.

Clostridium perfringens bacteria from foods left at room temperature, generally meat, poultry, stews, casseroles and gravy. Symptoms: abdominal pain and diarrhoea. Sometimes nausea and vomiting.

Enteroviruses, rotaviruses, parvoviruses from food and water contaminated by sewage, or careless food handling. Symptoms: severe diarrhoea, nausea and vomiting, plus respiratory symptoms.

Listeria monocytogenes bacteria from unpasteurized milk and cheese, raw and cooked seafood, and vegetables. Symptoms: similar to influenza; also fever.

Mycotoxins from moulds on beans and grains that have been stored in a moist place. May cause liver and/or kidney disease.

Salmonella bacteria (more than 2000 kinds) found in raw or undercooked meat, poultry, fish or eggs. Symptoms: abdominal cramps, diarrhoea, fever and vomiting.

Shigella bacteria found in poultry, milk and dairy products. Symptoms: abdominal pain, cramps, diarrhoea, fever, sometimes vomiting, and blood, pus or mucus in stools.

Staphylococcus aureus bacteria found in food left too long at room temperature: meats, poultry, fish, egg dishes, potato salad, cream-filled pastries. Symptoms: diarrhoea, vomiting, nausea, and abdominal cramps.

Yersina enterocolitica bacteria found in raw vegetables, meats, water and unpasteurized milk. Symptoms: fever, headache, nausea, diarrhoea and general malaise; mimics influenza.

In the UK, well over half of all food-borne illnesses are directly due to negligence in the home. You have little control over sanitation practices in cafes, snack bars, delicatessen and canteens, but make sure proper rules are followed in your own kitchen.

What you can do

- Always wash your hands after using the toilet.
- Keep everything in the kitchen *clean*.
- Shop carefully by observing the expiry dates printed on food labels.
- Most food poisons can be controlled by refrigeration and cooking. Keep cold foods COLD and hot foods HOT. Store tinned foods in a cool clean dry pantry, away from leaky pipes or seeping moisture.
- Cook food thoroughly, to destroy further growth of bacteria; refrigerate leftovers promptly.
- Keep pets, household cleaners and other chemicals away from food. Control household pests such as flies, rats, mice and cockroaches.
- On picnics or camping, never drink water taken from streams, rivers or ponds. Take bottled water for drinking, making tea or mixing with food.
- For worry-free picnics, place perishable food in an insulated, portable ice-chest, and keep the cooler in the shade.

To counteract poisonings if stomach upsets are severe, keep in stock two antidotes: 1) Syrup of ipecacuanha (ipecac), also known as Brazil root, and 2) Activated charcoal. Consult your chemist or doctor about dosage for children and adults, and be sure not to exceed the recommended dose.

What the doctor can do

The physician may use gastric lavage, or stomach pumping, by inserting a tube in the stomach, adding water or other liquids, and then sucking out the stomach contents.

Parasites and worms

Worm-induced diseases have fortunately become rare, thanks to better control of our water supply and sewage systems. They are not entirely gone, however, and occasionally some appear as epidemics where water or food has been contaminated, or food is insufficiently cooked; they can easily be picked up when you go abroad to developing countries. Children's swollen bellies in Third World countries indicate not only poor food, but also the many parasites that the children carry. Dr Otto Soemarwoto, Director of the Institute of Ecology in Bandung, estimates that 60 per cent of the population of Indonesia carry parasitic worms because human waste is dumped in the water supply.

Amoebic dysentry is caused by *Entamoeba histolytica*, which enters via the mouth from faeces-contaminated water, food and the environment. It causes attacks of diarrhoea over a prolonged period and may produce complications such as liver and lung abscesses. Diagnosis can be made when the organism is found in the stool.

Anisakiasis is transmitted to humans in raw or undercooked seafood, such as sushi, harbouring *anisakis* nematodes, a type of roundworm. Worms have been found in cod, mackerel and herring. In the Netherlands, most cases occur after the opening of the herring season. Symptoms can be confused with acute appendicitis, Crohn's disease, gastric ulcer or gastrointestinal cancer. Sometimes the parasite can be felt tingling in the throat.

Beef tapeworm enters in larva form from poorly cooked or raw infected beef. It produces abdominal distress and appendicitis-like symptoms. Diagnosis can be made when eggs are found in stool.

Fish tapeworm enters in larva form from infected freshwater fish, may cause pernicious anaemia or bowel obstruction. Immature eggs are found in the stool.

Giant intestinal roundworm eggs can enter intestines after eating contaminated vegetables, producing colic and diarrhoea. Immature eggs or worms are found in stools.

Giardia lamblia is a microscopic parasite that enters as a cyst through the mouth from water contaminated by human faeces. Giardia is now recognized as a world-wide scourge afflicting 2 to 10 per cent of the population in various countries. Even in developed countries where drinking water is chlorinated before distribution, giardia can escape routine disinfection. Filtration before chlorination is needed to rid water of the cysts. The infection produces mucous diarrhoea, abdominal cramps and weight loss.

Hookworm may enter via the mouth, but more commonly penetrates the soles of the feet from faeces-contaminated soil. The worm can cause stools to be darkened with blood pigments or mature eggs may be found in stool.

Schistosomiasis is caused by bathing in water infested with flukes that penetrate the skin and mature in about two months into adult worms that invade intestines or bladder.

Threadworm enters through the skin, usually the feet, from faecal contamination of soil. It causes diarrhoea and stomach pain. Larvae may be found in stools.

Trichinosis. This parasitic disease is caused from infection with the roundworm *Trichinella spiralis*, as a result of eating raw or undercooked pork, processed pork or pork products.

Visceral Larva Migrans is an infection with nematode larvae which are normal intestinal parasites of pet dogs and cats. If a child plays in soil or a sandbox contaminated by pet faeces containing parasite eggs, then transfers the eggs to his/her mouth while playing, the eggs hatch in the human intestine. Larvae can penetrate the intestinal wall, enter the bloodstream, and remain alive for months, producing damage as they move about. They can cause fever, coughing, liver enlargement and lung inflammation.

Whipworm, pinworm and **dwarf tapeworm** can enter as an egg through the mouth. The source is contaminated soil. They produce diarrhoea, nausea, and anaemia. Whipworm can sometimes cause acute appendicitis in children. Pinworms often affect an entire family.

What you can do

Prevention is better than cure. Never drink untreated surface water. Be sure that your sources of water and food are scrupulously clean and sanitary. Handle food carefully, after washing your hands. Store food carefully. Cook meat, fish and eggs thoroughly. Avoid recipes using raw fish or meat. Thoroughly wash all fruits and vegetables, especially those which have come into contact with soil. Cover pets' sandboxes when not in use, and don't let the children play in them. Pets should be de-wormed regularly by a veterinarian. Do not walk with bare feet, especially when in developing countries.

What the doctor can do
If worms or parasites are evident or suspected, the physician can examine stool samples and prescribe effective medications or special enemas in some cases. If the worm is in the stomach, examination and removal can be done without surgery. If it is in the intestine, surgical removal is the only available treatment at present.

Inflammatory Bowel Disease

There are other mysterious diseases that attack the bowel wall, causing chronic intestinal inflammation. These bewildering and stubborn illnesses of unknown cause are called *inflammatory bowel disease* (IBD).

Inflammatory bowel disease is the name given to a group of chronic digestive diseases of the small and large intestines. Your doctor may refer to your particular condition by any one of several terms, including *colitis, proctitis, enteritis,* and *ileitis.* Doctors often divide IBD into two groups: *ulcerative colitis* and *Crohn's disease.*

Ulcerative colitis causes ulcers and inflammation of the inner mucous membrane (mucosa) lining the colon. Inflammation nearly always begins at the rectum and spreads back through the colon. The lining becomes fragile, filled with blood, bleeds easily, and usually causes bloody diarrhoea. When inflammation involves the whole colon, there may be fever, muscle aches, heavy sweating and poor appetite.

Crohn's disease (named after Burrill Crohn, MD who de-scribed it in a paper in 1932) is an inflammation that extends into the deeper layers of the intestinal wall. The disease is usually limited to the ileum (ileitis) or involves both the ileum and upper colon (ileocolitis). When Crohn's disease is confined to the colon, it is referred to as Crohn's colitis. Sometimes inflamma-tion may also affect the mouth, oesophagus, stomach, duo-denum, appendix or anus.

Both ulcerative colitis and Crohn's disease are chronic conditions and may recur over a lifetime, but many people will have long periods – sometimes years – when they will be free of symptoms.

What are the symptoms of IBD? The most common symptoms are diarrhoea and abdominal pain. Ulcerative colitis usually causes rectal bleeding as well. Crohn's disease may also cause rectal bleeding, but less often than ulcerative colitis does. In either disease, inflammation, fever and bleeding may be serious and persistent, leading to weight loss and anaemia. Children may also suffer stunted growth and delayed development. In Crohn's, the first signs often show up at the anus: haemorrhoids, unhealing cracks and fistulas. Onset tends to be gradual, so Crohn's may go unnoticed for years.

What causes IBD? There are many theories about what causes IBD, but none has been proven yet. The current leading theory suggests that some infectious or toxic substance, possibly a virus or bacterium, interacts with the body's own immune defence system to trigger an inflammatory reaction in the intestinal wall. A new species of *Mycobacterium* has been identified in the intestines of some Crohn's disease patients. Although there is much scientific evidence that people with IBD have abnormalities of the immune system, doctors do not know whether these abnormalities are a cause or a result of the disease. Doctors do believe, however, that Crohn's disease and ulcerative colitis are *not* caused by emotional distress, tension, anxiety, other psychological disorders, or the result of an unhappy childhood.

How common is IBD? The number of people who get Crohn's disease, after increasing steadily for the past thirty years, appears to have reached a plateau. Hitherto, the incidence has been highest in the British Isles, Northwestern Europe, Scandinavia and North America. In recent years, however, researchers have observed an increase in frequency in developing nations throughout the rest of the world, and doctors cannot yet explain why.

Men and women are affected about equally, but some people seem to be more likely targets for these diseases. IBD is more prevalent among whites than blacks, Orientals, Hispanics or American Indians, although no population group is immune from attack. Jews are significantly more affected than Gentiles, except curiously in Israel where rates are not high. Jews who do have it in Israel are predominantly from a European or American background (*Ashkenazim*) and not from Middle East countries (*Sephardim*).

IBD has two peaks in age of onset. Although IBD can begin at any age, there is a concentration of cases between the ages of 12 and 28; between ages 50 and 60, there is a second wave of new cases. When children get IBD, they are apt to be more severely affected than adults, and their disease is often more widespread: conditions such as fever, anaemia or joint complications tend to be more evident, and slowed growth and delayed sexual maturity are often problems. Often failure of normal growth is the first sign of trouble and is noted before other symptoms begin.

Does IBD run in families? About 25 per cent of people with Crohn's disease or ulcerative colitis have a blood relative with some form of IBD – most often a brother or sister, and sometimes a parent or child. It is not yet known whether this tendency is due primarily to heredity or to environment. When patients with IBD are considering having children, the normal course of pregnancy and delivery is not usually affected by the presence of IBD in the mother, and most pregnancies result in normal children.

What you can do
Although no special diet has been proven effective in preventing or relieving IBD, some people find it easier to tolerate a diet that avoids milk, hot spices, fibrous foods and alcohol. When milk is a problem, drink milk substitutes, predigested milk, or commercially available lactase which is added to milk. It is more important to maintain good general nutrition and adequate caloric intake rather than emphasize or avoid any particular food. Large doses of vitamins may produce harmful side effects. Emotional upsets can aggravate any illness, so reduce the stress in your life. Get enough exercise and rest. At the onset of an attack, remain in bed for a few days. A hot-water bottle or electric heating pad can relieve abdominal cramps.

What the doctor can do
The doctor will examine your rectum with a proctoscope or sigmoidoscope, obtain a culture of a stool, and want you to have a barium enema X-ray. Your physician can prescribe drugs, not

as a cure, but for the relief of abdominal cramps and diarrhoea. *Sulphasalazine* often lessens the inflammation of ulcerative colitis, but the drug shouldn't be used by anyone sensitive to sulphites. More serious cases may need cortisone-type medicine, such as *prednisone* and *prednisolone*.

Your doctor may recommend nutritional supplements of special high-calorie liquid formulas, especially for youngsters with growth retardation produced by IBD. A small number of patients may need periods of intravenous feeding in order to rest their bowels, or for those whose bowels cannot absorb enough nourishment from normal food taken by mouth.

Ulcerative colitis can be permanently cured by surgery. About one-third of patients eventually need the removal of the colon and rectum: a small opening (*stoma*) is made in the front of the abdominal wall and the tip of the lower small intestine, the ileum, is then brought through. The stoma is fitted with a pouch to collect waste products, and this external opening to the intestine is called an *ileostomy*.

Crohn's disease can be helped by surgery, but not cured by it. The inflammation tends to return to sites in the intestine immediately next to the area that has been removed . About two-thirds of Crohn's disease patients require surgery, however, to provide relief from chronic disability or to correct complications.

Dangerous conditions may arise when severe ulcerative colitis progresses rapidly, with deep growth of ulceration in the bowel wall. In such cases, there may be paralysis and swelling of the colon (*acute toxic dilation*) and rectal bleeding. Leakage of the colon's contents into the abdominal cavity (*perforation*) may cause inflammation of the lining of the abdominal cavity (*peritonitis*). These uncommon problems often require surgery.

If ulcerative colitis is widespread throughout the colon, and lasts for many years, patients may be at increased risk of cancer of the colon or rectum. See your doctor for regular colon examinations.

Crohn's disease affects deeper layers of the bowel wall than those affected by ulcerative colitis, often involving the small intestine but sparing the rectum. Although rectal bleeding is less common in Crohn's, the disease tends to thicken the bowel wall with swelling and fibrous scar tissue, and the bowel may become narrowed (*stenosis*), which can result in intestinal obstruction or 'blockage'. Crohn's disease may also cause deep ulcer tracts (*fistulas*) that burrow all the way through the bowel wall into surrounding tissues, into adjacent segments of the intestine, or into other nearby organs such as the urinary bladder or vagina. These abnormal tunnels between inflamed intestine and adjoining tissues are marked by pain or difficulty in urinating, or by passing blood, gas or faeces with the urine or through the vagina. Fistulas are a common complication of Crohn's disease often associated with pockets of infection or abscesses in the anus and rectum, and are a means of diagnosing Crohn's disease. They can sometimes be treated with medication, but in many cases they must be drained surgically.

Irritable Bowel Syndrome

Not to be confused with ulcerative colitis is irritable bowel syndrome (IBS), a disorder of the colon's *contractions*. It is sometimes called spastic colon or mucous colitis, but colitis is a misnomer since it implies inflammation, of which there is none with IBS. Although often causing considerable discomfort, IBS does not cause inflammation, has no relationship to ulcerative colitis, has not been shown to lead to serious illnesses such as Inflammatory Bowel Disease, and there is no evidence that IBS is a precursor of cancer of the colon. A person can have IBD and IBS at the same time.

Doctors don't yet know what causes irritable bowel syndrome, but they do know that symptoms seem to be triggered by stress, that women with the syndrome outnumber men three to one, and whites more often than blacks.

There are two major types of IBS: one has the major symptoms of gas, abdominal pain, diarrhoea or constipation, or alternating bouts of both; excess mucus may appear in the stools. The other type of IBS causes urgent diarrhoea first thing in the morning, during meals, or afterwards. The physical symptoms are often accompanied by fatigue, depression and anxiety; many victims are tense and anxious, with hurried irregular meals and overwork. But IBS is not purely psychological. It is associated with the muscles of the bowel which, instead of contracting three times a minute, may contract up to nine times a minute, stretching the intestinal wall and creating pain.

What you can do

You can control IBS in two ways: by diet and by managing stress. Avoid the foods you find irritating, and reduce consumption of fatty foods that stimulate excessive contractions of the bowel muscles; protein, on the other hand, may decrease contractions. Peppermint tea or capsules of peppermint oil are thought to produce relaxation of bowel muscles – although peppermint can also induce heartburn, if you are a susceptible. A high-fibre diet may help.

Regular vigorous exercise can help in the management of stress because it releases opiate-like brain chemicals, *endorphins*, which lessen anxiety. You can also help the bowel by certain types of exercise such as curl-ups which, when you bend back and forth, also bend your colon and provoke normal intestinal contractions instead of spasms.

Please realize that IBS is extremely common, not caused by disease, and although uncomfortable, it is not serious.

What the doctor can do

When abdominal pain, diarrhoea and constipation become intolerable, talk with your doctor. Irritable colon can imitate more serious intestinal conditions, so it is wise to have a doctor's examination to rule out other diseases.

Diverticulosis and Diverticulitis

Some physicians believe there may be an association between chronic IBS and *diverticulosis*. The word *diverticulum* (plural, *diverticula*) means a pocket, and diverticulosis is a condition in which dozens of small out-pouchings or sacs (diverticula) balloon out at weak points in the wall of the colon, wherever blood vessels supplying nutrition and oxygen merge with the bowel. Diverticula occur mostly in the sigmoid colon because this section is the narrowest and the contents are more solid, but they can also be scattered along the transverse colon. The size of diverticula can range from 6mm to 25mm (¼ inch to 1 inch).

Diverticulosis is common in developed Western societies, affecting between 30 and 40 per cent of people over the age of

50, and the majority of people over 60 or 70 years. The condition affects men more than women, and is generally caused by a diet with too little 'roughage'. A low-fibre diet produces small-volume stools, and to move such stools along, the colon must clamp down harder. Excessive clamping down leads to high pressures within the bowel which may account for the pushing out of the pouches.

Diverticulosis itself produces no symptoms and most people wouldn't know if they had diverticula unless an X-ray were taken, as only 15 per cent of people with diverticulosis develop complications such as *diverticulitis*, bleeding or perforation. The condition is called diverticulitis when the diverticula become inflamed, infected and develop an abscess or boil. Pressure in the colon caused by straining can make a tiny hole (perforation) in a diverticulum where bacteria or faeces can become trapped, creating infection and pain from peritonitis – a medical emergency. Where perforation extends to penetrate the urinary bladder, the connection is a *fistula*, and causes urinary tract infections.

Diverticulitis is sometimes referred to as '*left*-sided appendicitis' because the pain in the lower abdomen is similar to that of the *right*-sided pain of appendicitis. The pain from diverticulitis may last minutes, hours or days, appearing at any time without relation to eating. Other symptoms may include abdominal swelling, nausea, vomiting occasionally, fever and malaise.

What you can do
Increase the fibre in your diet. Do this gradually, to avoid bloating, flatulence or other discomfort. A high-fibre diet widens the colon slightly, and reduces the pressure. During acute attacks of diverticulitis, have a liquid diet and get bed rest.

What the doctor can do
Your physician may prescribe an antibiotic to combat the infection. In a severe case, a hospital stay may be necessary for intravenous feeding in order to put the bowel at rest. If peritonitis or fistulas develop, the doctor will perform repair surgery. If severe attacks recur, the physician may remove the portion of intestine that contains the pouches, and rejoin the intestine to enable normal bowel function to resume.

CHAPTER 11

Other serious problems

Bleeding

This is a symptom of digestive problems rather than a disease in itself. It can occur as the result of a number of different conditions, many of which may not be life-threatening, but which should not be ignored. The most common cause for bleeding is probably haemorrhoids, but the anal area may also be the site of cuts (fissures) in the lining, inflammation or tumours. Bleeding can originate anywhere in the digestive system (see Table 9).

Bleeding from an inflammation at the lower end of the oesophagus can be caused by acid or bile. Enlarged veins (varices) at the lower end of the oesophagus may rupture and bleed massively. Cirrhosis of the liver is the most common cause of varices.

The stomach is a common site of bleeding. Alcohol, aspirin, aspirin-containing compounds, and various drugs (particularly those used for arthritis) can cause individual ulcers or gastritis. 'Stress ulcers' can result after burns, shock, head injuries or cancer, or after extensive surgery. Bleeding can occur from benign tumours or cancer, although these disorders do not usually cause massive bleeding.

The small intestine is not a common source of bleeding, except for ulcers in the duodenum. In adults, the most common cause of bleeding from the small intestine, other than duodenal ulcers, is Crohn's disease.

The large intestine and rectum are common sites of bleeding. Benign growths or polyps of the colon are common and are thought to be forerunners of cancer. These growths can cause

TABLE 9

BLEEDING IN THE DIGESTIVE TRACT

Site	Possible problem	Colour of blood in stool
Oesophagus	Inflammation (oesophagitis) Enlarged veins (varices)	black
Stomach	Ulcers Inflammation (gastritis)	black
Small intestine	Duodenal ulcer Crohn's disease	dark red or black
Large intestine and rectum	Haemorrhoids Inflammation (ulcerative colitis) Diverticulitis Colorectal polyps Colorectal cancer	bright red

Note: Bleeding may be occult (hidden), producing no change in stool colour.

either bright red blood or occult bleeding. Colorectal cancer usually causes bleeding at some time. Inflammation from many causes can produce extensive bleeding from the colon. Various types of intestinal infections can cause inflammation and bloody diarrhoea. Ulcerative colitis can produce extensive surface bleeding from tiny ulcerations. Crohn's disease of the large intestine can produce spotty bleeding. Diverticula of the colon can result, rarely, in massive bleeding. And as one gets older, abnormalities may develop in the blood vessels of the large intestine and may result in recurrent bleeding.

What genetic factors lead to bleeding? A variety of genetic disorders may be responsible for bleeding in the digestive tract. Certain types of cancers may tend to run in families. Some benign growths that involve the small and large intestines, such as those seen in familial polyposis are clearly hereditary. Also hereditary blood vessel disorders may lead to frequent bleeding in the digestive tract. Finally there are inherited clotting disorders, such as haemophilia, that can cause bleeding anywhere in the body, with the gastrointestinal tract being a common site.

Many lifestyle factors can contribute to diseases that produce bleeding in the digestive tract: alcohol, drugs, infectious agents and stress. Tobacco and coffee may interfere with the healing of peptic ulcers and may therefore be indirectly responsible for bleeding. Low-fibre diets are associated with diverticulitis.

If massive bleeding occurs suddenly, there may be weakness, dizziness, faintess, shortness of breath, abdominal cramps and diarrhoea. Shock may occur, with a rapid pulse, drop in blood pressure, pallor and difficulty in producing urine. With slow chronic bleeding, there may be a gradual onset of fatigue, lethargy, shortness of breath, and pallor from anaemia.

What you can do
Cut out smoking, drinking alcohol, and taking aspirin. Note any changes in bowel habits, consistency and colour of stool (whether the colour is black or red). Iron supplements or foods such as beetroot can give stool the same appearance as bleeding in the digestive tract. If blood does occur in stools, consult your doctor without delay.

What the doctor can do
A stool sample will be tested for blood content (a *Guaiac test*) and a blood sample will be checked for signs of anaemia. The site for bleeding may be diagnosed by a fibre-optic endoscope or a barium X-ray. Endoscopy can view the location of the problem, take tissue biopsies and colour pictures. Radioactive scanning may be used for locating sites of bleeding in the lower tract.

To prevent or reverse shock from extensive bleeding, your doctor may ask you to stay in hospital for a blood transfusion.

Haemorrhoids

Each of us has veins around the anus that tend to stretch under pressure, similar to varicose veins in the legs. They act like inflatable cushions, forming a tight seal that prevents stool from leaking from the rectum. One set of veins is inside the rectum (internal), and another is under the skin around the anus (external). Sometimes the veins over-inflate and become *haemorrhoids*, also known as 'piles'.

Humans develop haemorrhoids because of their upright posture, heredity, occupation, diet and cultural patterns. Conditions can be triggered by constipation, diarrhoea, pregnancy, infection of the anus and rectal cancer. As a rule, they do not cause pain or bleeding, but problems can occur when these veins become swollen. Increased pressure can come from straining at bowel movements and chronic constipation which pushes out veins, sitting too long on the toilet, or from other factors such as coughing or sneezing, lifting heavy objects, obesity or liver disease. They are a common problem among people who have to stand or sit for long periods such as bus, taxi and lorry drivers.

There appears to be a genetic susceptibility to haemorrhoids and varicose veins that makes these problems very common. About half of people under the age of fifty have haemorrhoids to some extent. Women may begin the development of haemorrhoids during pregnancy as the pressure of the foetus and

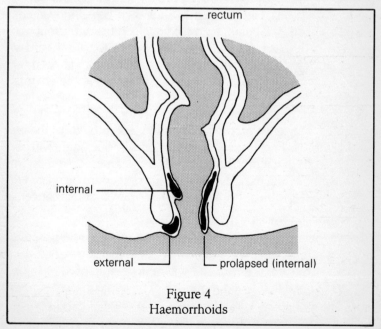

Figure 4
Haemorrhoids

hormonal changes cause haemorrhoidal veins to enlarge. These veins are also placed under severe pressure during the birth of the baby, but for most women such haemorrhoids are only temporary and disappear after delivery.

The only symptom you may notice of internal haemorrhoids is bright red blood on toilet paper or in the toilet bowl. Sometimes, however, these internal veins stretch and may even fall down (*prolapse*) through the anus to the outside of the body (*protruding haemorrhoids*). See Figure 4.

Veins around the anus cause problems when blood clots form in them, and they become large and painful; these are called *thrombosed external haemorrhoids*.

What you can do

An ounce of prevention . . . Often all that is needed to reduce symptoms is to include more fibre in your diet to soften stools. Drinking six to eight glasses of liquids (not alcohol, and not too much milk) each day will also help. And be active: move around, walk, exercise, to help move stools through your body. Pass bowel movements as soon as you have the urge. Don't sit on the toilet too long; the longer you sit, the longer pressure is put on the haemorrhoids. Cleanse gently after each bowel movement.

For haemorrhoidal pain, try a cold pack on the anus, followed by a sitz bath (sitting in warm water) three or four times a day. Apply zinc oxide ointment or powder, or petroleum jelly, to the area. Medicated suppositories are also available at the chemist or pharmacy.

It is imperative to see your doctor, however, any time you have bleeding, seepage, protrusion, prolapsed and thrombosed haemorrhoids. Rectal bleeding, with or without pain, with or without signs of haemorrhoids, needs proper medical attention. Persistent bleeding may lead to anaemia or it could be related to other serious problems such as polyps or even colon cancer.

What the doctor can do

Your physician will examine the anus and rectum, and possibly give a barium X-ray to rule out cancer or some other disease of the digestive system. The doctor will remove prolapsed haemorrhoids or those that bleed too much. The surgeon may simply put a rubber band around the base of the vein to cut off circulation, and the haemorrhoid withers away within a few days.

Sometimes a chemical is injected around the vein to shrink it. Other methods include the use of freezing (*cryosurgery*), electrical or laser heat, or infrared light to destroy haemorrhoidal tissue.

Intestinal Polyps

Polyps and cancer of the rectum can cause a type of bleeding similar to haemorrhoids. Intestinal polyps, or abnormal growths in the mucous surface of the colon, are believed to be precursors of colorectal cancer. All *true* polyps – the most common type – are *adenomatous* (those having glandular cell structures) and should be surgically removed as a preventive measure. They are found most often in the rectum and the sigmoid colon. *False* or *Pseudopolyps* are not growths (so far as is known), but are areas where inflamed tissue has accumulated; they are seen in people with Inflammatory Bowel Disease. *Inflammatory* polyps do not become malignant, but a small percentage may be malignant from the start.

The most frequent symptoms are painless rectal bleeding or the passage of mucus. They are most often found during routine examinations of the intestines or if an examination is being made for some other purpose.

Familial polyposis is a rare inherited condition: if members of your family have developed large numbers of polyps in the intestine, you are more likely to develop these lumps also. If you belong to a high-risk family, you should have your doctor examine your gastrointestinal tract regularly.

What the doctor can do
If a polyp is within 20cm (8 inches) of the rectal opening, the doctor will remove it with a sigmoidoscope through the rectum. With improved techniques of colonoscopy, almost any polyp with a 'stalk' can be removed through a colonoscope, by ensnaring with a wire loop, or cauterizing and removing. The removed polyp will be examined to make sure it is not cancerous. If cancer is found, the segment of the bowel where it grew must also be removed.

Cancer of the Colon, Rectum, Small Intestine and Anus

Symptoms of these cancers are blood in the stool (either bright red or black), changes in bowel habits, such as constipation or diarrhoea, abdominal discomfort and pain, a burning sensation when urinating, vomiting, or a feeling of a lump or mass in the abdomen.

Colon and rectal cancer

This progresses in stages: early cancer affects the membrane of the first layer of colon-rectal tissue; then the mucosa or submucosa; the tumour then spreads through the wall of the intestine, to the lymph nodes and on to other distant sites such as the liver.

This type of cancer can run in families, and where there is a family history of rectal polyps, ulcerative colitis, or a diet heavy in smoked, pickled or salted foods. Many cancers of the large bowel develop because people have a susceptibility gene and then are exposed to other environmental factors such as high-fat, high-protein, low-fibre foods typical of most urban industrialized countries. Colorectal cancer occurs more frequently in Britain, Western Europe, the United States, Australia and New Zealand, than in Japan, Africa, and most of the developing Third World countries.

Cancer of the small intestine

This is much less common than those of the oesophagus, stomach, pancreas and colon; it is almost always treatable and sometimes curable. *Adenocarcinomas* are the most common and usually show up as bowel obstructions; *lymphomas* also obstruct the bowel and have symptoms of bleeding; and *leiomyosarcomas* produce bleeding, obstruction, weight loss, fever and abdominal pain, and may reach large size before diagnosis.

Cancer of the anus

This condition is uncommon. It is a highly treatable, often curable cancer. The stage of the cancer is important in determining the first treatment, which is usually surgery, radiation and chemotherapy.

What you can do
The less time that food takes to move through the colon, there is less chance that toxins and cancer-causing substances make contact with the bowel lining: have a wholesome, balanced diet that is low in fat, moderate in meat, but plenty of fibrous foods such as fresh unpeeled fruits, fresh vegetables, wholegrain breads and cereals. Carrots, and vegetables in the cabbage family are particularly good.

What the doctor can do
Diagnosis by your doctor can include a digital examination of the rectum, direct viewing of the rectum and colon with a colono-scope, the use of X-ray examinations, barium X-rays, and a Guaiac test of stools for traces of blood.

Surgical removal is the primary treatment for colon and rectal cancers. If enough normal colon remains, the surgeon will rejoin healthy sections so that normal colon function is resumed. When this is not possible, a *colostomy* may be necessary following surgery, depending on the location and extent of the cancer, to provide an opening between the colon and the abdominal wall, to permit elimination of body wastes.

Resources

United Kingdom:

Action for Smoking and Health (ASH), 5-11 Mortimer Street, London W1N 7RH (telephone: (071) 637 9843)

Alcoholics Anonymous, P.O. Box 1, Stonebow House, Stonebow, York YO1 2NJ (telephone: (0904) 644026)

Anorexia Bulimia Nervosa Association, Tottenham Women and Health Centre Annexe, Tottenham, London N15 4RX (telephone: (081) 885 3935)

Association for the Study of Obesity, 50 Ruby Road, London E17 4RF

British Association of Cancer United Patients, 121-123 Charterhouse Street, London EC1M 6AA (telephone: (071) 608 1785)

Ileostomy Association of Great Britain and Ireland, Amblehurst House, Chobham, Woking GU24 8PZ (telephone: (09905) 8277)

Institute for the Study of Drug Dependence, 1-4 Hatton Place, London EC1N 8WD

National Association for Colitis and Crohn's Disease, 98A London Road, St. Albans AL1 1NX (telephone: (0727) 44296)

Release, (for drug dependence) 169 Commercial Street, London E1 3BW (telephone: (071) 377 5905)

Weight Watchers (UK) Ltd, 11 Faircress Estate, Dedworth Road, Windsor SL4 4UY (telephone: (0753) 856751)

World Organization of Gastroenterology, Dept of Medicine, Ninewells Hospital, Dundee DD1 9SY

United States:

Alcoholics Anonymous World Services, General Service Office, P.O. Box 459, Grand Central Station, New York, NY 10163 (telephone: (212) 686 1100)

American Digestive Disease Society, 7720 Wisconsin Avenue, Bethesda, MD 20814 (telephone: (301) 652 9293)

American Hepatitis Association, 30 E.40th Street, Room 305, New York, NY 10016 (telephone: (212) 599 5070)

American Institute of Stress, 124 Park Avenue, Yonkers, NY 10703 (telephone: (914) 963 1200)

Center for Ulcer Research and Education Foundation, 11661 San Vincente Boulevard, Suite 304, Los Angeles, CA 90049 (telephone: (213) 825 5091)

Gluten Intolerance Group of North America, P.O. Box 23053, Seattle, WA 98102 (telephone: (206) 325 6980)

Narcotics Anonymous, P.O. Box 9999, Van Nuys, CA 91409 (telephone hotline: (818) 997 3822)

National Association of Anorexia Nervosa and Associated Disorders, Box 7, Highland Park, IL 60035 (telephone: (312) 831 3438)

National Clearinghouse for Drug Abuse Information, P.O. Box 416, Kensington, MD 20895 (telephone: (301) 443 6500)

National Council on Alcoholism, 1511 K Street NW, Washington, DC 20005 (telephone: (202) 737 8122)

National Digestive Diseases Information Clearinghouse, Box NDDIC, Bethesda, MD 20892 (telephone: (301) 468 6344)

National Foundation for Ileitis and Colitis, 444 Park Avenue South, New York, NY 10016 (telephone: (212) 685 3440)

National Ulcer Foundation, 675 Main Street, Melrose, MA 02176 (telephone: (617) 665 6210)

Overeaters Anonymous, P.O. Box 92870, Los Angeles, CA 90009 (telephone: (213) 542 8363)

Smoking and Health – Center for Disease Control, Dept. of Health and Human Services, 5600 Fishers Lane, Rockville, MD 20857 (telephone: (301) 443 1575)

Australia:

Alcohol and Drug Information Service (telephone: in Sydney 331 2111; outside Sydney 008 42 2599 toll free)

Alcoholics Anonymous, 127 Edwin St. North, Croydon, NSW (telephone: 02 700 1000)

Cancer Information and Support Society, 65 Bay Road, Waverton 2060 (telephone: 922 2334)

Coeliac Society, 10 Diana Avenue, West Pymble 2073 (telephone: 498 2593)

Colostomy Association, 630 George St., Sydney 2000 (telephone: 264 2741)

Selected references

Arora, David. *Mushrooms Demystified*. (Berkeley, California: Ten Speed Press, 1979)

Billington, B.P. 'Observations from New South Wales on the Changing Incidence of Gastric Ulcer in Australia'. *Gut* 6:121 (1969)

Brodibb, A. and D. Humphreys. 'Diverticular Disease: Three Studies'. *British Medical Journal* 1:424-25 (1976)

Burrow, Gerard N. and Thomas F. Ferris. *Medical Complications during Pregnancy*. (Philadelphia, PA: W.B. Saunders Company, 1988)

Coffey, Wayne. *Straight Talk About Drinking*. (New York: New American Library, 1988)

Eisenberg, M. Michael. *Ulcers* (New York: Random House, Inc., 1978)

Gear, J. et al. 'Symptomless Diverticular Disease and Intake of Dietary Fibre'. *Lancet* 1: 511-14 (1979)

Gonvers, J.J. 'Tabagisme et Gastro-enterologie'. *Therapeutische Umschau* 40(2): 139-142 (1983)

Heimlich, H.J., K.A. Hoffman, and F.R. Canestri. 'Food-choking and Drowning Deaths prevented by External Subdiaphragmatic Compression'. *Annals of Thoracic Surgery* 20: 188 (1975)

Heimlich, H.J. 'A Life-saving Maneuver to prevent Food-choking'. *Journal American Medical Association* 234: 398 (1975)

Helferich, William and Dennis Westhoff. *All About Yogurt*. (Englewood Cliffs, NJ: Prentice-Hall, Inc. 1980)

Kikendall, J.W. et al. 'Effect of Cigarette Smoking on Gastro-intestinal Physiology and Non-neoplastic Digestive Disease'. *Journal of Clinical Gastroenterology* 6(1): 65-79 (February 1984)

Konturek, S.J. et al. 'Effects of Nicotine on Gastrointestinal Secretions'. *Gastroenterology* 60(6): 1098-1105 (June 1971)

Lampe, Kenneth F. and Mary Ann McCann. *AMA Handbook of Poisonous and Injurious Plants*. (Chicago, IL: American Medical Association, 1985)

Morra, Marion and Eve Potts. *Choices: Realistic Alternatives in Cancer Treatment*. (New York: Avon Books, 1987)

Mott, Lawrie and Karen Snyder. *Pesticide Alert*. (San Francisco: Sierra Club Books, 1987)

National Foundation for Ileitis and Colitis. *The Crohn's Disease and Ulcerative Colitis Fact Book*. (New York: Charles Scribner's Sons, 1983)

Royal College of General Practitioners. 'Oral Contraceptive Study'. *Lancet* 2:957 (1982)

Scragg, R.K.R., A.J. Michael and R.F. Seamark. 'Oral Contraceptives, Pregnancy and Endogenous Oestrogen in Gallstone Disease'. *British Medical Journal* 288:1795 (1984)

Seitz, H.K. et al. 'Alkohol und Karzinogenese'. *Leber Magen Darm* 12(3): 95-107 (1982)

Short, A.R. 'The Causation of Appendicitis'. *British Journal of Surgery* 8:86 (1920)

Singh, D.S. 'Smoking and Disorders of the Gastrointestinal Tract'. *Indian Journal of Public Health* 19(2): 74-78 (April-June 1975)

Stewart, D.N. and D.M. de R. Winser. 'Incidence of Perforated Peptic Ulcer: Effect of Heavy Air Raids'. *Lancet* 1:259 (1942)

Turnberg, L.A. 'Coffee and the Gastrointestinal Tract'. *Gastroenterology* 75 (1978)

Tyler, Varro E. *The Honest Herbal*. (Philadelphia, PA: George F. Stickly Company, 1981)

Wald, A. et al. 'Effect of Caffeine on the Human Small Intestine'. *Gastroenterology* 71: 738-42 (1976)

Ward, Ritchie R. *The Living Clocks*. (New York: Alfred A. Knopf, Inc., 1971)

Whong, W.Z. et al. 'Formation of Bacterial Mutagens from the Reaction of Chewing Tobacco with Nitrite'. *Mutation Research* 158(3): 105-110 (1985)

Index